Welcome Back!

This book is for those seeking expert guidance on how to rebound and thrive again after the pandemic lockdowns.

Welcome Back! will empower you to systematically use science-based diagnostics and techniques to repair, recover, and renew your health, physically and mentally, after the traumatic events we've all experienced because of COVID-19.

Dr. Elaine Chin, a trailblazer in integrative personalized wellness, engages people to take control of their health by being proactive, with a preventive focus, to achieve optimal health and well-being.

Welcome Back!

How to Reboot Your Physical and Mental Well-Being for a Post-Pandemic World

DR. ELAINE CHIN

SUTHERLAND
HOUSE
TORONTO, 2021

Sutherland House
416 Moore Ave., Suite 205
Toronto, ON M4G 1C9

First edition, September 2021

If you are interested in inviting one of our authors to a live event or
media appearance, please contact publicity@sutherlandhousebooks.com
and visit our website at sutherlandhousebooks.com for more
information about our authors and their schedules.

Manufactured in Canada
Cover designed by Lena Yang
Book composed by Karl Hunt

Library and Archives Canada Cataloguing in Publication
Title: Welcome back! : how to reboot your physical and
mental well-being for a post-pandemic world / Dr. Elaine Chin.
Names: Chin, Elaine, 1964- author.
Identifiers: Canadiana 2021022651X | ISBN 9781989555477 (softcover)
Subjects: LCSH: Self-care, Health. | LCSH: Mental health. |
LCSH: Well-being. | LCSH: COVID-19 Pandemic, 2020——Health aspects. |
LCSH: COVID-19 Pandemic, 2020——Psychological aspects.
Classification: LCC RA776.95 .C45 2021 | DDC 613—dc23

ISBN 978-1-989555-47-7

Contents

CONTENTS

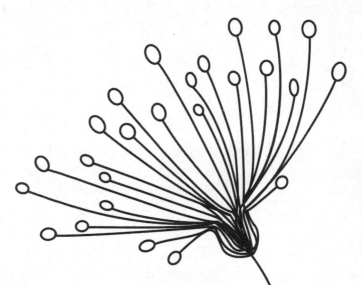

When this book's manuscript was submitted to the publisher, more than 153 million people worldwide had officially contracted COVID-19 and recovered. Tragically, more than 3.5 million people globally had died of the disease.[1] However, every person on planet Earth has been in many ways impacted by this pandemic. Let's help each other, repair our bodies and minds, recover our relationships with family and friends, and find a way forward to thrive with a renewed sense of health resiliency.

This book is dedicated to those who have died of COVID-19 and to the families who have lost them.

May we honor them by pledging that we will treasure our life, live it to its fullest in the best way we can, full of health and vitality.

Never again will we take our well-being for granted.

Introduction

"10-9-8-7-6-5-4-3-2-1!
Happy New Year and Welcome to 2020!"

As the New York City crystal ball in Times Square ignited and the fire-works lit up the sky, I was excited to see a new decade begin. For a doctor, "20/20" means perfect vision. And I was hopeful that the next decade would bring on joy and personal growth. Yet another chance to hope for better things to come.

But what unfolded could never have been predicted, making what the Queen of England said about the year 1992 – "annus horribilis" – seem like an overexaggeration today. What a profoundly humbling experience we all endured in 2020. The world shared a story of its peoples suffering together, burying their loved ones not in the hundreds, but in the hundreds of thousands. Yet there was hope for better days to come, ending the year with the arrival of multiple vaccines, distributed first in wealthier countries.

Ugly inequalities were brought out into the spotlight in 2020. People we took for granted before became critical workers who provided our basics for daily survival. From packaging hand sanitizer shipments to bagging our groceries to protecting and saving our lives without recognition, these workers finally became "appreciated." We called them our frontline and essential workers, and yet today, there continues to be a forgotten subcommunity of invisible frontline workers who are taking care of our vulnerable communities – they're still struggling to get the appropriate supports. Our elderly, new immigrants, refugees, homeless people, and those with mental illness, including drug addicts, have also been significantly impacted too. These groups are dying in higher numbers compared to their broader communities.

The year was filled with so much news that it could have been spread out over one decade, but the updates were impossible to ignore with lockdowns and everyone staring at their TV and social media feeds. They were world-changing, paradigm-altering stories. You could not avoid hearing news about the coronavirus, Black Lives Matter, Trumpism, apocalyptic wildfires, Russian cyber-hacking, and epidemic business bankruptcies and unemployment.

Because you are reading this book, you survived the first few waves of the COVID-19 pandemic. You were not alone in feeling the fear, anxiety, grief, and loss. All of us have experienced physical and mental health effects after being under the pandemic cloud and rounds of lockdown.

Welcome Back! will put the power of achieving optimal health back in your hands by getting you onto a path of recovery and developing physical and mental resiliency against future illnesses. This book provides you with a science-based guide based on healing the body and mind in a step-wise repair, recovery, and renewal model.

> Together we must come out of this grotesque experience with a better perspective, that *without health, we have nothing. Literally nothing.*

We've missed out on so much and realized we took for granted our family gatherings, having a job to physically go to (rather than zooming in our bedrooms or basements), seeing and collaborating with colleagues in 3D, teachers being able to nurture our kids in person (rather than through a screen), celebrating graduations, attending weddings and funerals, attending our houses of worship, sharing a glass of wine with friends at a table at our favorite local restaurant (no more Styrofoam takeout), and getting on a train, bus, or airplane to explore the world.

I am excited to share my personal journey with you today. My life was broken open in 2020, but it also set me free to explore who I was and what I want to become. In the pages that follow, you'll learn how to rebound from the lockdowns caused by the pandemic and be more physically and mentally resilient, thriving as a whole person.

"Turn your wounds into wisdom."[2]

— *Oprah Winfrey*

During difficult times, we are forced to learn more about ourselves and others. COVID-19 has forced us to self-reflect as we sit at home during lockdowns. We have been facing adversity, but we can overcome it. Hopefully, we can learn from it.

Pathway to Renewed Resiliency

Healthcare systems around the world have been pushed to the limits as we struggle through the greatest health crisis of our generation. We have listened to many experts and public health leaders, who try to offer their best advice. But as the science and data change, they make new recommendations that conflict with the previous insights. Vast amounts of misinformation in our social media sphere and political agendas adds confusion to this mix, often clashing with the science.

No wonder many of us are confused, anxious, and, frankly, frustrated. Many of us have now tuned out because we are exhausted about all things COVID-19.

But don't give up on what to do next.

As a personalized medicine physician, I've spent my life helping people take a holistic, preventive approach to their health and well-being. Allow me to help you sort through and process the science, and offer you an easy pathway to immunity from COVID-19. More importantly, you can learn to reduce your stress and anxiety and thrive both physically and mentally.

Perhaps you've received science's gift to humankind for 2020/21, a COVID-19 vaccine. This shot marks the beginning of the end of this

COVID-19 nightmare for everyone. Here are three simple beginning steps to take back control of your health and life.

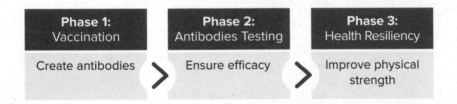

Phase 1: Get Your COVID-19 Vaccinations

On December 8, 2020, the first Oxford/AstraZeneca vaccine was given to a grandmother in England, followed soon after with the first Pfizer-BioNTech vaccine administered to a retired nurse in the United States. Different countries and territories are embracing various approaches for rolling out the vaccine – who should get the vaccine first and what should the timing be for the second shot? All of us have become exhausted trying to keep informed. Here's a summary of our current vaccine insights at the time this book went to the publisher (last updated April 20, 2021):

- All the vaccines currently available are generally both safe and effective in preventing severe illness and death due to the wild type (original strain) of COVID-19.
- There are concerns around the AstraZeneca vaccine regarding the risk of blood clots, though rare. It seems to occur in only certain people with thrombocytopenia (low platelets).[3]
- During the clinical research for the vaccines, the second injection (the booster) was scheduled for around 21 to 30 days, allowing for the rapid completion of the clinical trials. Recent clinical evidence suggests that waiting beyond the 21 days (Pfizer) and the 30 days (Moderna and AstraZeneca) provides sufficient continued protection with only the first injection.
- New variants of concern (VOCs) contain mutations from the wild type (original strain), which increase the virus's contagiousness, lethality, and, possibly, resistance.

- More boosters will likely be required in the future to manage new VOCs.

Definition: Vaccine

A vaccine is a substance that stimulates a person's immune response against a specific bacteria or virus – without having to endure the actual virus or bacteria.

Should you be exposed to the disease at a later date, your body recognizes the infectious agent and produces antibodies to attack and neutralize it, protecting you from developing serious symptoms.

Phase 2: Test for Post-Vaccination Antibodies Against COVID-19

Studies now suggest that antibodies are still present in your body at least 6 to 12 months post-vaccination. What determines the efficacy of your post-vaccination immunity?

- The quantity of antibodies your body produces to fight the wild and variant strains
- The efficacy of your antibodies to bind to the virus and neutralize the wild and variant stains

A post-vaccination antibodies test can reduce your anxiety and concerns about your level of resistance against the SARS-CoV-2 virus causing COVID-19. Furthermore, new research suggests the vaccine has an efficacy of 50% even if it induces antibody levels 80% lower than those found, on average, in a person who has recovered from COVID-19.[4]

If you reply positively to these four questions, you will be able to more confidently reclaim your social freedoms and safely reengage in life as you knew it before the pandemic hit.

1. Did you make any antibodies? Let's get tested.

Note: Some people do not mount as strong an antibody response after a vaccination, especially those who are elderly or immunocompromised.

2. Do you have enough antibodies? Let's do a count.
   Note: Although your test might detect antibodies, it's critical to make sure you have a high quantity of them.

3. Are your antibodies effective against the SARS-CoV-2 virus? Let's test their strength.
   Note: Laboratory testing can determine the strength of your antibodies by assessing their ability to bind tightly to the virus and neutralize it.

4. Will your antibodies work against the new SARS-CoV-2 variant strains? Let's test their efficacy.
   Note: Through avidity and pseudovirus-neutralization testing, you will discover the efficacy of your antibodies based on the best of what science knows today.

Second Generation Antibodies Testing

Using a small blood sample, this post-vaccination antibody laboratory-based test helps determine if your immune system has developed antibodies after natural infection or vaccination against the SARS-CoV-2 virus spike protein.

You can perform this test yourself using a self-test kit to collect a few drops of blood and send it to the laboratory* for processing. This test has been shown to be equally sensitive and reliable when compared to a standard blood test.

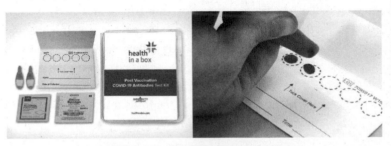

Available at: covidimmunitypassport.com

And if you discover that your immunity response is suboptimal overall or not strong against some variants, it's not the end of the world. In fact, it's manageable because you now know your risks. Continue to wear your mask and maintain social distance until you can get a booster shot. Your physician will be able to best advise you on next steps.

Phase 3: Boost Your Health Resiliency

The COVID-19 pandemic has triggered a major paradigm shift when it comes to our healthcare. It has taught us that although our healthcare system was there for us pre-pandemic, we now need to become more informed about all aspects of our health, be proactive, and take charge of our personal well-being.

Knowing your health numbers is a great place to begin. It allows you to manage disease risks by improving your lifestyle. COVID-19 has been a wake-up call for all of us. For many, it's prompted a fresh look at the possibilities that science and technology hold for a more personalized medicine approach to our wellness. Advances in science and technology are changing every single facet of health and wellness.

The future is patient-centric and data-driven, and connecting those dots is critical so that we can make an earlier diagnosis, improve treatments, and enhance our quality of life.

For me, as a doctor, it's about equipping you with the information you will need to respond to the medical and wellness challenges you will face.

Before the pandemic, I embarked on an important initiative, Health-in-a-Box (www.healthinabox.com), which leverages the success of my practice at Executive Health Centre. It is a virtual healthcare offering that makes personalized medicine accessible to everyone by taking advantage of do-it-yourself, point-of-care diagnostics that can be acted upon. The antibodies test for post-COVID-19 vaccination is one of many examples that I will share with you in this book.

Although I've not been part of the frontline team of doctors saving lives in the ICU, I'm here for you on the sidelines as your health coach and to help you set your path forward to reduce your anxiety, repair your body and mind, and recover your life with family and friends. It's time to *Welcome Back!* everyone into our lives and thrive with a renewed sense of health resiliency.

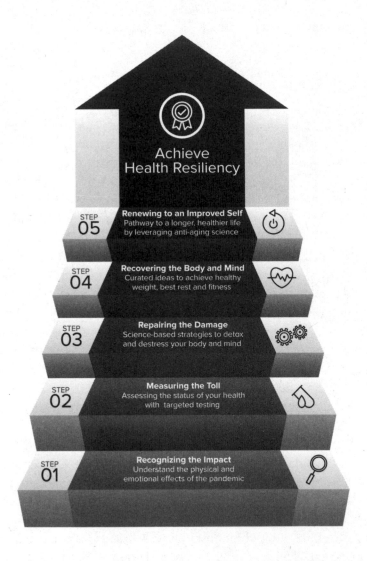

Achieve Health Resiliency

STEP 05 — **Renewing to an Improved Self** — Pathway to a longer, healthier life by leveraging anti-aging science

STEP 04 — **Recovering the Body and Mind** — Curated ideas to achieve healthy weight, best rest and fitness

STEP 03 — **Repairing the Damage** — Science-based strategies to detox and destress your body and mind

STEP 02 — **Measuring the Toll** — Assessing the status of your health with targeted testing

STEP 01 — **Recognizing the Impact** — Understand the physical and emotional effects of the pandemic

Pathway to Health Resiliency

Section 1: The Impact of Lockdown

Recognizing the physical and emotional effects of the pandemic

Section 2: Assessing the Toll

Measuring the status of your health with targeted testing

Section 3: Repairing the Damage

Science-based strategies to detox and de-stress your body and mind

Section 4: Recovering the Body and Mind

Curated ideas to achieve healthy weight, best rest, and fitness

Section 5: Renewing to an Improved Self

Pathway to a longer, healthier life by leveraging antiaging science

THE IMPACT OF LOCKDOWN

CHAPTER 1

A Tale of Two Coronaviruses

Origin Story

It was November 2003. Yet another respiratory infection was noted in China. Certainly, no one appeared to be fussed about it. In late February 2003, a woman returned from Hong Kong to Toronto with flu-like symptoms. She died 10 days later at home while under the care of her family. A few days afterward, her 44-year-old son went to the ER with a high fever, severe cough, and difficulty breathing. He was treated with Ventolin and sent home. Days later, he returned to the hospital and went to the ICU with suspected tuberculosis and was put in isolation. He died on March 13. We did not know it yet, but the first pandemic of the 21st century was taking hold, right in Toronto.[5]

The family members who visited him in the ICU also had symptoms and were all later admitted.

And the nurse who took care of him in the ER on his first visit to the hospital also infected two other patients, who later died, one in a different hospital. It turned out these two patients, directly and indirectly, infected almost a hundred people, including in-hospital patients, hospital workers, first responders, and family members related to these close-contact cases.

They named the infection SARS (severe acute respiratory syndrome).

There was no test available at that time, just a cluster of symptoms to identify and a look at associated contacts and travel history.

By March 25, Health Canada reported 19 cases of SARS in Canada (18 in Ontario and one case in Vancouver). But 48 patients with a presumptive diagnosis of SARS were admitted to hospital by the end of that day.

The Ontario government declared SARS a provincial emergency on March 26, 2003. Under the Emergency Management Act, the government has the power to direct and control local governments and facilities to ensure that necessary services are provided. All hospitals in the Greater Toronto Area (GTA) and Simcoe County activated their Code Orange. Four days later, provincial officials extended access restrictions to all Ontario hospitals.

Code Orange

Impacted hospitals suspended all nonessential services, limited visitors, created isolation units for potential SARS patients, and provided protective clothing and equipment (such as gowns, masks, and goggles) for staff.

New protocols and policies were developed to manage this new kind of infection. Hospital teams developed a communication system – dial-in conference calls – so they could share up-to-the-minute information with other teams. A command structure was put in place within all hospitals across Canada to deal with this new pandemic. Physical access to hospitals was limited to a single entrance. Nonessential workers were told to stay at home. Visitors were not allowed, with some exceptions. Surgical procedures and outpatient appointments were canceled. "Work quarantine" also was imposed: health workers were asked to travel directly between work and home without using public transit and without stopping at any other destinations.

Those who had visited certain hospitals during specific time periods were asked to self-isolate. Schools took a hard stance of zero tolerance for cases. At one high school, 1,700 students were quarantined after only one student became ill. More than 13,000 Toronto residents voluntarily complied with quarantine.

On May 14, 2003, the World Health Organization (WHO) removed Toronto from the list of areas with recent local transmission. The outbreak had come to an end. In total, Canada logged 140 probable and 178 suspect infections. Twenty-four Canadians had died, all from Ontario. SARS was the first identified strain of the coronavirus species, a viral respiratory disease of zoonotic origin (a pathogen that has jumped from a nonhuman animal to a human). It was formally named SARS-CoV-1.[6]

SARS Toronto: Phases I and II	Phase	
	I	II
Exposure	No. (%)	No. (%)
2002	91 (33%)	52 (42%)
Hospital (worker, patient, visitor)	49 (18%)	64 (51%)
Other health care (clinic, EMS)	8 (2.9%)	2 (1.6%)
Household contact	76 (28%)	9 (7.2%)
"Community"	16 (5.9%)	---
Travel	12 (4.4%)	---
Under investigation	21 (7.7%)	---

"The experience with SARS in Toronto indicates that this disease is entirely driven by exposure to infected individuals. Transmission occurred primarily within health care settings or in circumstances where close contacts occurred. The infectious agent was spread by respiratory droplets in the great majority of cases, and some patients were more infectious than others. Ultimately, the strict adherence to precautions – and practice implementing them – was critical to the containment of SARS in Toronto and the restoration of safe conditions for hospital staff and patients."[7]

— *Donald E. Low, M.D., FRCPC, Canadian microbiologist noted for his role in battling the SARS outbreak of 2003*

2003: My Battle with SARS (SARS-CoV-1)

In March 2003, my then-husband was a physician working at a SARS-designated hospital in Toronto, at St. Michael's Hospital. I had a family practice office located inside the Trillium Health Centre, Mississauga site, another hot spot for patients admitted with SARS.

As the situation progressed and new insights came to light hour by hour, we had to decide on the fly at work and at home. As a family, we made life-altering decisions day by day. It happened so fast. Within a month of the first case in Toronto, the province went into a state of emergency.

At Trillium, screeners wearing full gowns and gloves took our temperature at the front entrance. We showed them our ID badges and responded to a set of questions before being allowed into the hospital. Patients were admitted only for immediate medical conditions. Moms gave birth to babies without their spouses around. Family and visitors were not permitted in the hospital.

My clinic was near the front door, where people were screened. The glass protected me from the outside, yet I was reminded that we were not fooling around for hours every day. The virus was deadly, and who was next? As case counts went up and people died, we were oddly thankful, each day, that it wasn't a colleague who was taking care of the SARS patients.

At no point in the outbreak was there a discussion about a shortage of appropriate personal protective equipment (PPE). As usual, all of us who needed masks, gloves, and gowns had access to them.

At the time, we had a 4-year-old son. We kept him home from pre-school because he was in a high-risk home. We self-isolated in the house. My husband ate by himself and slept in a separate room each night for months. And yes, we updated our wills. I stopped working after my hospital locked down hard in April, when cases jumped. Only essential staff were allowed into the hospital. I stayed away from work and told our nanny to stay at her own house to keep her safe.

My husband and I didn't see our parents. Mine were elderly and frail. His parents and brother were all in healthcare settings. We didn't mingle with them either, to reduce the risk of family-community spread.

As each week progressed, there seemed to be more information about how this virus spread; it was highly contagious and deadly, and it killed fast. But it seemed under control inside hospitals and in the community.

The day-to-day nightmare in 2003 seemed to be a nonstop roller coaster with a 24–7 sense of fear. The SARS outbreak ended in 6 months – relatively short, in retrospect. Thankfully, it didn't progress to a global pandemic. And then, suddenly, life went back to normal.

SARS 2020: Wave 1

In early January 2020, a news story appeared that mimicked many others before it. Like other viral-infections stories, this article out of China reported a few pneumonia cases that seemed to worry the Chinese government.[8] The WHO outlined there was a mysterious pneumonia sickening dozens in the country. The last respiratory virus pandemic had been the swine flu (H1N1), in 2009, and we managed to get that under control quickly. Although there had been lots of infections, there was a relatively low death rate. And like the SARS virus pandemic (SARS-CoV-1) of 2003, H1N1 hit hard but fast in Asia and Canada, and then it was gone. With aspirational hopes for 2020, I was cautiously optimistic that history was on our side and that all would be well soon.

> The virus appeared to be "over there" and "not here." *But we were so wrong!*

In 2020, things went from bad to really "*$#%$" bad; no words can adequately describe the year's horrific trajectory. Here's a simple chronology of the first 3 months of the COVID-19 (SARS-CoV-2) virus[9]:

- January 11: China reports the first novel coronavirus death.
- January 21: The first case is confirmed in the United States.
- January 23: China imposes a strict lockdown in Wuhan and begins constructing two hospitals (completed on February 2).
- January 25: A Toronto man who had recently traveled to Wuhan, China, and his wife are confirmed as the first two cases in Canada.

- January 28: Health officials in British Columbia say a man in his 40s is presumed to have the new coronavirus and is doing well as he recovers at his Vancouver home.
- January 30: WHO declares a global health emergency.
- February 5: The Diamond Princess cruise ship quarantines in Japan.
- February 11: The novel coronavirus is renamed COVID-19.
- February 26: The first case of suspected local transmission is confirmed in the United States.
- February 29: The first COVID-19 death is reported in the United States.
- March 3: The Centers for Disease Control and Prevention (CDC) lifts restrictions for virus testing.
- March 13: Trump declares a national emergency in the United States.
- March 15: The CDC warns against large gatherings.
- March 17: The coronavirus is now present in all 50 states of the United States.
- March 17: Northern Californians ordered to "shelter in place."
- March 18: China reports no new local infections.
- March 18: Canada shuts the border to non-Canadian citizens.
- March 19: Italy's death toll surpasses China's.
- March 20: New York City is declared the U.S. outbreak epicenter.
- March 24: Japan postpones the Olympics.
- March 24: India announces a 21-day complete lockdown.
- March 26: The United States leads the world in COVID-19 cases.
- April 2: Global cases hit one million.

And then, as they say, the rest is history, as we lived through it locally – one lockdown at a time.

What made my hair stand up on end was not the fact that we had "officially" one death in Wuhan on January 11, but that the infection had so quickly spread to other continents thanks to the relatively new norm of global and intercontinental travel. Sequentially, in less than 2 weeks, Italy announced their first death due to the novel coronavirus, and by January 21 and 25, the United States and Canada, respectively, announced their first cases.

2020: My Battle with COVID-19 (SARS-CoV-2)

Until January 25, when the first two cases of novel coronavirus were announced in Canada, I had been on standby mode, hoping it would not happen to us so soon. And it was in Toronto, the city where I live. I realized the virus was moving as fast as the nonstop flights to and from China and Europe could fly and land in Canada.

I learned early on in SARS that despite the assurances by WHO and other public health officials, what we see on the ground lags by days and is relayed to the public in a controlled and deliberate manner. And this became ever so true for my experiences in 2020. I learned not to trust the official version of the unfolding events.

I called up my expert colleagues in my global community and determined that this novel coronavirus was a real global threat. The virus was "nasty," said a colleague on the Danish COVID-19 advisory panel, and only time would tell how bad it would become. This time, a virus was not going to get the upper hand in my life, messing with my patients and my family.

> I went into fight mode as if my life and the lives of those around me depended on it. And it turned out not to be too far from the truth.

The next day, I sent out my first blog to my clients about the virus:

January 26, 2020. Bulletin #1: How Novel Coronavirus Impacts You

Considering the fact that the first coronavirus case was diagnosed in Toronto, Canada, our team felt it would be helpful to communicate with you to provide some data points, plus what you can do to protect yourself.

It is our team's view that the epidemic in China has yet to peak and that there will likely be more cases outside of China, including in Canada. This is a normal exponential-curve phenomenon. Cases reported thus far in the United States and other countries were all connected to individuals who had recently traveled from Wuhan. The next wave will be those who infect others outside of the epicenter.

We all need to stay vigilant given the reality of global travel and the highly contagious person-to-person infection characteristic of this virus.

All of us who lived in Toronto during SARS in 2003 can recall how disruptive and, quite frankly, scary it was for those of us who worked in hospitals at the time. I do believe that we are more prepared today as a global community.

- *Communication systems exist now which didn't at the time when SARS began.*
- *The public health departments and hospitals are more prepared, with protocols and stocked-up equipment in place.*
- *DNA testing now allows us to identify the coronavirus within 24 hours.*

All these technologies make for an improved response today. We are not functioning in a 'black box' for weeks, when there was a time, we simply did not know who was really sick with the SARS virus and how the virus was behaving.

Here are a few more insights so you can do some proactive planning. What we know so far:

- *A sudden surge of respiratory illnesses was first identified in Wuhan in December 2019, with presentations greatly resembling viral pneumonia.*
- *The virus identified appeared to be similar to SARS but seemed "less deadly." Signs and symptoms of this illness include fever, cough, and difficulty breathing.*
- *Evidence so far indicates a human-to-human transmission for this virus, with an incubation period of about 3 to 5 days.*
- *Those with weakened immune systems and those with a history of chronic conditions are at higher risk of complications, if infected.*
- *You're more likely to get a cold or seasonal flu, especially if you've not taken this year's effective flu shot. You might want to do so if you haven't yet done so.*
- *This year's flu shot will NOT protect you from getting this coronavirus infection.*
- *The Pneumovax vaccine will NOT protect you from getting viral pneumonia, as it combats only specific types of bacterial pneumonias.*

- *No antiviral treatment for coronavirus infection has been proven to be effective so far.*

Recommendations:

As of today, the risk level remains at Alert Level 3 from the U.S. Centers for Disease Control and Prevention (CDC); the alert was issued on Tuesday January 22nd.

"Avoid Nonessential Travel to Wuhan, Hubei Province, China, for the Novel (new) Coronavirus."

I encourage all of you to consider postponing all travel to China at this time, given the uncertainty about how rapidly the virus is spreading, as well as the possibility of travel disruptions due to new areas in China that are under quarantine. Given it's also Chinese New Year period, all business activities are also mostly shutdown.

Assuming we can all avoid travel to China, here are my general guidelines (which should be truly followed year-round!):

- *Avoid traveling when sick (traveling with a fever from an unrelated condition could result in increased screenings and other travel issues).*
- *Stay home and don't go to work to infect others. Encourage those around you who are also sick to stay home, including your staff.*
- *Avoid close contact with people suffering from acute respiratory infections. Walk away from them.*
- *Practice good hygiene through frequent handwashing, especially after direct contact with sick people or their environment, and after touching public items (such as being in trade shows). Use hand sanitizers.*

Consider the following when traveling from home for business:

- *Wear gloves – don't touch things that are not your personal items – it's easier in winter now.*
- *Have your own hand sanitizer gel and use it OFTEN when in public.*
- *Bring Lysol-type wipes with you and use several of them to WIPE*

DOWN your entire airplane area, including the table, touch screen, armrest, headrest, etc.

- *Bring a face mask – you never know when you might sit near someone sickaAvoid getting the general cold or flu as it can lower you're the strength of our immune system and make you more susceptible to getting the coronavirus.*
- *Yes, wipe down your hotel room, especially the TV clicker and electronics you use in the room.*

Lifestyle:

- *Get your sleep – 7 to 8 hours ideally.*
- *Keep doing your exercise if you are feeling well (don't exercise if you are sick with a cold).*
- *Eat lots of fruits and vegetables and avoid too much sugar; it's also a good time to be "drier" on the alcohol side of the leger.*
- *Consider taking supplements that offer more immunity protection in addition to the standard antioxidants zinc, B-complex, and elderberry.*
- *We often recommend AHCC (active hexose correlated compound, a potent antioxidant), which can be used to protect or rescue those who get frequent colds and flus.*

I trust the health community has learned big lessons from the SARS outbreak and we are far more prepared and organized to make sure it doesn't spread in Canada. Take care. We should be fine this time around. Let's hope.

I was planning to travel with caution to visit my son, who was attending Northwestern University in Chicago, a big international airport hub on January 30. It was ahead of his 21st birthday and Chinese New Year. While I thought of canceling the trip, I decided to go ahead because I had a few mother-doctor things to do "for him" and his roommate – two guys learning to live on their own!

As many parents know, FaceTime is nice for "how are you?" chats with your kids, but I needed to have a serious face-to-face talk with him about my deep worries for his safety around this virus and how to use his PPE. I brought it to him in person to show him how to make the masks snug, take gloves off safely, and secure the face shield on tightly. Last but not least, I wanted to get him "stocked up" before the lockdown I anticipated (which did happen on campus), with a run-on for food and, yes, toilet paper too.

Time to Play Offense, Not Defense

By early February, stories about the virus seemed to be unfolding in an out-of-control manner, like a badly written reality TV show. The storyline was getting repetitive and uglier by the day.

It started in China, and spread to Italy, and then the apocalyptic tragedies began in North America too.

[10]CNBC HEADLINE:

China is building two hospitals in less than 2 weeks to combat coronavirus

The Chinese city of Wuhan is scrambling to complete construction on two hospitals that will treat coronavirus victims, according to state media.

The outbreak has killed 213 people and infected nearly 10,000.

Construction began last week on the two temporary hospitals, which will provide 2,600 beds.

This was not the first time the Chinese government had built a hospital in 2 weeks. The last time was in Beijing in 2003 to deal with the SARS virus. And now they were building *not one, but two* hospitals. While most people were watching the build-out in abstract amazement of the engineering feat (which was truly impressive), I was saying to myself, *OMG, this is really bad, the virus is out of control in Wuhan, whether they admit it on state television or not.* The situation was dire enough for the central government to step in and mandate a build-out, which meant they knew something we didn't. But it was clearly in front of us to see. Check out the video on YouTube (www.youtube.com/watch?v=53nhErXUd9A), as it is an architectural feat in itself.

At first, I was unrealistically hopeful to see the cases were limited to northern Italy and were sporadic, like we had in Toronto during SARS. But soon reality set in.

By February 27, public health officials in Canada reported 33 confirmed cases of the novel coronavirus, with 20 cases reported in Ontario, 12 in British Columbia, and one in Quebec.

On February 27, I sent out my second blog about the virus.

February 27, 2020. Bulletin #2: Scare Yourself to Health

Here we are on February 27, 2020, 1 month since I sent out a note to my patients about the "new" coronavirus. Since then, I've now lost count of where there are new cases and how many of them are in each country. While professional agencies around the world have not yet called it a pandemic (which has huge economic implications), academically and practically we are there.

It's worldwide and highly contagious, and a large portion of the population is infected.

The good news for now is: COVID-19 presently has a 3% mortality rate – mainly hitting those who have a chronic illness or are elderly (in other words, a weakened immune system).

Some epidemiology models are showing that 65% of the population will become infected with COVID-19. Let's hope it doesn't come true. A vaccine won't be commercially available for at least 1 year.

By February 29, the first cluster, or outbreak, of the novo-coronavirus cases were confirmed at the Life Care Center of Kirkland, a nursing facility outside of Seattle, Washington. The CDC reported 27 of the 108 residents, and 25 of the 180 staff, had some symptoms.[11]

Cruise ships were proving to be very vulnerable too. The 2,666 passengers of the Diamond Princess cruise ship, for example, were forced to quarantine at the Yokohama port in Japan on February 3. The virus infected the passengers quickly. By February 23, 691 cases of the novo-coronavirus disease were confirmed.[12]

And on March 6, the Grand Princess cruise ship was forced to dock in Oakland, California. Forty-five people aboard were experiencing respiratory symptoms and were tested; 46.7% of these, including 19 crew and two passengers, tested positive.[13]

Confirmed cases onboard continued to increase and passengers who were showing symptoms were not allowed to dock. Then-president Donald Trump wanted "to keep the numbers down in America."[14]

And so the misinformation and lies began, starting at the top, in America.

Early American Reaction

"It's going to disappear. One day – it's like a miracle – it will disappear. And from our shores, we – you know, it could get worse before it gets better. It could maybe go away. We'll see what happens. Nobody really knows."

— Former president Donald Trump, February 27, 2020

Mass testing was not available in the United States in March 2020. The CDC failed to create their own coronavirus testing kits.[15] Without testing, tracing, and isolating, the virus took hold, and Americans were doomed to become very sick, very quickly.

What's more, Americans were still allowed to travel globally and domestically in spring 2020.

Then came Italy. Towns of people were dying, and it seemed they could not stop it. They pleaded for masks, gowns, gloves. Surely this was just a delivery delay and not a procurement supply issue? How can they be short of PPE? Italy has a good healthcare system and is a G7 country. They can get this under control.

On March 21, Italy reported 793 new coronavirus deaths, a one-day record that saw the country's toll shoot up to 4,825 – 38.3% of the world's total. The total number of fatalities in the northern Lombardy regions around Milan was more than 3,000 by March 20.

Early Canadian Reaction

Canada, too, had few novo-coronavirus tests available, but thankfully the nation's case counts early in the pandemic were relatively low, likely due to stay-at-home restrictions. Early in the pandemic, labs completed only 827 tests between March 27 and April 30. The positivity rate was at 0.4%.

Between May 26 and 31, only 1,061 tests were performed but the positivity rate had risen to 1.4%.

Testing was ramped up to 7,014 tests, with a steady positivity rate of 1.1%. This was followed by a relatively calm summer before the second wave hit Canada in the fall.[16]

I believe the low overall infection rate during Wave 1 in Canada can be attributed to the fact that Canadians followed public health guidelines and because the Canada–U.S. border was closed to nonessential travel effective March 18.

Preparing for the Worst

In early March, I committed to three highly focused goals recognizing this virus was not only a medical crisis but a business crisis too, and it has a global impact.

1. Preserve personal health and safety.
2. Access critical PPE for staff, patients, and our families.
3. Test for novel coronavirus infections.

> In a frenzy of fear and determination, I set out to manage this virus. And to not have it manage me.

I realized early on that China's exports would come to a halt if China went into a complete lockdown as a country. Of immediate concern to me was that all the raw materials for medicines and supplements came from there.

I urgently asked my patients to renew their supply of medications. If we could run out of toilet paper, then certain drugs were at risk too.

I renewed their prescriptions for 6 months. Those who did not heed my ask ended up having to go month to month with their medications, caused by pharmacy rationing during the first lockdown.

Other critical supplements important for immune health – including antioxidants such as active hexose correlated compound (AHCC), vitamin C, vitamin D, and anti-inflammatory omega fatty acids – were also at risk. (Learn more about these supplements in Chapter 4.) We ordered a significant supply of key supplements for the office to dispense to our patients. (The inventory went dry soon after, in April.)

Also in early March, one of my patients discovered she had cancer and needed radiation and chemotherapy. Because her immune system would be weakened with treatment, I wanted to set her up with supplies. It should have been simple to find a few N95 masks – the most effective type of mask for protection from COVID-19. I contacted my regular medical supplier, and they simply said, "We don't have any in stock. No delivery date available." Really?

I simply needed a single box of masks and couldn't find one. What I soon came to realize was that there was no inventory to be had.

Everyone was after masks. Hospitals, nursing homes, and governments too. It turned out no one had stockpiled for a rainy day! The just-in-time inventory model doesn't work during a global pandemic. My desire for a box of medical-grade masks morphed into trying to get the provincial governments of Ontario and British Columbia and the federal government of Canada as many as five million of them.

By mid-March, I was immersed in the world of global piracy, with the Americans against the world. Naively, I thought getting a few cartons of masks wouldn't be a problem. It seemed so easy for my medical supplier and friend Manny Kapur when we somehow managed to secure five million masks. It was straightforward. Find a friend, put down a deposit, and the shipment would come in a few weeks. We wondered out loud why the Canadian government had had so much trouble procuring PPE and had come back from China many times with either fake or damaged PPE – and, once, an empty cargo plane. I would soon learn a lesson about global trade.

What happened when five million medical masks for Canada's COVID-19 fight were hijacked in China

NATIONAL✦POST

"The stuff was at the airport ready to be shipped. We had it on the tarmac," said Manny Kapur. "Then the craziest thing happened."

Author of the article:
Adrian Humphreys

Publication date:
Apr 17, 2020

Dr. Elaine Chin and Manny Kapur had their order for five million medical masks to fight COVID-19 but they were hijacked on the tarmac at an airport in China by someone willing to pay four times the price.

In a desperate bid in early March to get medical masks for the fight against COVID-19, a Toronto doctor and her friend arranged for five million masks to be shipped directly from a manufacturer in China. They took out a line of credit to pay the deposit as their masks spun off the line and were packed for Canada.

Dr. Elaine Chin and Manny Kapur closed the deal and made arrangements, including working with Canada's federal and provincial governments in Ontario and B.C.

"The stuff was at the airport ready to be shipped," said Kapur. "We had it on the tarmac. I was hearing on the news about companies bringing in 10,000 masks, 5,000 masks – and we had five million masks coming.

"Then the craziest thing happened."

Their shipment disappeared at Shanghai airport.

"We never got the shipment onto the airplane," Chin said. "It turns out we were suddenly outbid."

At the airport, a surprise and sudden offer four times the agreed price short-circuited their deal, they were told.

"To this day I have no idea where that shipment went," Kapur said. "It's like somebody pulled up with a truck, picked up our pallets and put them on a different plane and it disappeared, and nobody will know because it was just cash changing hands.

"It was like the Wild West at the airport."

To Chin, it sounded like "modern-day pirates."

The panicked buying from governments and institutions around the world not only highlights the frenzy to secure protective equipment as the pandemic spread, but also the determination and generosity that rose to meet it.

Chin and Kapur never got those masks, but they did create a campaign that is raising funds for the COVID-19 fight.

Chin isn't on the front lines of COVID-19 treatment, but she and her then-husband were during the SARS outbreak in 2003. As she watched the novel coronavirus pandemic spread, it rekindled her fear. She is now the medical director of Toronto's Executive Health Centre and wanted to help.

At the same time, she had a patient with cancer whose aggressive treatments compromised her immune system. Chin wanted to give her surgical masks to protect her. Chin asked Kapur, who runs Xthetica, a wellness supply company, if he could get her patient a box of masks.

He made some calls and found they were already in short supply. He called a medical supply contact in Europe who told him they were ordering masks from China. He could do that too, he was told, but there was a minimum order.

He called Chin: "I can't get you one mask, but I think I can get you two million."

They had the beautiful audacity to try.

A few friends and clients donated and the two tapped personal lines of credit to make the down payment of US$500,000 for five million N95-equivalent masks.

They had their order confirmed on March 18. It was set to arrive March 23, Kapur said.

Government ministers and health officials took a keen interest when Chin and Kapur reached out about its importation; they started taking calls from federal, Ontario and B.C. ministers and officials who offered help, they said. Unexpected questions started: who was confirming the shipment hadn't been replaced with counterfeit gear? Who was supervising it at the airport? Was there an armed escort?

Meanwhile, Chin and Kapur were lining up private donors to buy the masks and then donate them to hospitals to bypass the bureaucracy of purchasing procurement.

"It was all working out just fine. Then it all blew up in the ether," Chin said. "We came to a standstill. It was heartbreaking, but we didn't give up."

When she broke the news of the hijacked shipment to her biggest donors, they suggested she find another way to use the money to help in the fight, Chin said.

She did.

Through the University of Toronto's Faculty of Medicine, from where she graduated, she started Masking Together Challenge, which is raising funds to support three elements in the COVID-19 fight.

They are still working to provide personal protective equipment for health-care providers, just probably not from China, and added two other outlets for help: funding accommodations for medical trainees who need to isolate from family, and for research into the novel coronavirus research and COVID-19.

Chin said the Challenge is designed to meet immediate and long-range goals.

"We need to make sure there is a safe sanctuary for residents and interns and fellows who are on the front line and still making student wages," she said.

"The pandemic is an unprecedented event on a global scale. We need to dig deep and think about solutions, and how we can each do our part.

"We started with looking for masks, but it is all about protecting each other from COVID-19."

The Untold Story

For days, I had been working with my friend Manny to call up my contacts in governments to see if they needed some help to access KN95 masks (which I soon learned were N95 equivalents in Asia and Europe), because it appeared we could get access to five million from Manny's friend, a buyer in Europe. It would be part of a side order to the 30 million she was ordering for Europe. We had to come up with a deposit and made a personal decision to dip into our personal lines of credit to get this rolling for the good of Canadians. Our families and even my clients (whom I also asked for support) thought we were crazy, but we felt it was time for us to step up. This was how we could help "the cause."

As the days rolled by, an agent of the British Columbia provincial government, who was himself a physician, called us to give support to securing the load of masks in China. The Government of Canada had "boots on the ground" and wanted to ensure we were getting bona fide medical-grade masks and would provide security in a Canadian warehouse at the airport. Air Canada would fly this cargo back on their government-chartered plane at no additional costs to us as these masks were mainly for Canadians. Was this real? I couldn't believe my ears. The inventory was being escorted by government agents? I realized then that we were playing in another league. In fact, five million masks equaled $5 million. We were not properly insured to lose these masks. This procurement game had truly become too big for us.

We were told the agents would check the mask inventory at the airport before boarding. But something happened in the hours leading up to the delivery. Trump had said the day prior that he would sweep across the globe to get the PPE for Americans, and he did. It turns out, Russia had offered to pay double the price to our European contact, but the Chinese suppliers told our European agent that it would take four times the price to get the supply of masks back. The game became too rich for us. We got out of the bidding war. Really big money was taking over. The cargo plane came back to Canada empty, yet again.

Also unforeseen was the lack of other medical supplies critical to fight the pandemic. Masks were just the beginning. Gloves, gowns, needles, regents to run genetics tests, and those cotton swabs to do the viral DNA tests were nowhere to be found. Guess who made most of these supplies? China.

I spent the following weeks trying to stay ahead of the sup-ply-chain curve.

What was unbelievable to the MBA half of my business psyche was that we had arrived at this place as a global community. Never did I think the world would have a shortage of lifesaving PPE inventory and resort to predatory practices. The virus triggered not only a global pandemic but also economic warfare of a sort that figuratively blew my mind. Medical supplies became a national security issue related to the well-being and safety of citizens around the world – and China held the balance? We got used to the cheap and easy-to-get goods from China without a thought to our national sovereignty.

As April approached, we found other suppliers for masks, gloves, face shields, gowns, and hand sanitizers. Some were thankfully being manufactured locally in Canada.

But I was extremely angry that our COVID-19 testing was in abysmal shape, not much better than the Americans. The lineups were long and the criteria to qualify for a test were ridiculous. This was unacceptable. We should have been able to test anyone who thought they needed one or anyone who was asymptomatic but in contact with a person who had tested positive for COVID-19. The gold standard was the Korean approach: setting up drive-by and walk-by booths for testing.

A colleague of mine who was advising the Danish government told me that one confidential German government study showed that less than 10% of one township was positive with antibodies, which meant that 10% of the township had COVID-19. But, astoundingly, of those with antibodies, more than 40% had been asymptomatic! Early signs of this reality can be seen from the Grand Princess cruise ship's testing swabs. The authors of a study who researched the infection rates concluded, "Asymptomatic patients with COVID-19 were more prevalent than those exhibiting symptoms and are an infection reservoir." Almost 50% of the passengers who tested positive remained completely asymptomatic.[17]

Untold Fact #1: Scientists knew that the novo-coronavirus could be spread unknowingly by a high number of asymptomatic people, but no public health agency said anything.[18]

Untold Fact #2: The virus was spreading in Europe in 2019, well before the pandemic was announced. Retrospective testing of blood and respiratory samples in Europe showed the virus was likely in Italy by September and in France by December. *Wow.*[19] [20]

So did my patients who were so sick in December and January have COVID-19 too? They were business travelers, and the airport was their second home. And by taking care of them, did I get it too? They made many visits back to my office for follow-up on persistent symptoms of fever, aches, and cough.

The answer lay in learning about our antibody status for COVID-19. Early on, the testing options available around the world were like the Wild West. Hundreds of different tests were approved by various countries, causing confusion and inconsistent interpretations of results. The Food and Drug Administration (FDA) in the United States allowed hundreds of unregulated tests to flood their market between April and June, while Health Canada approved only one.

I found no private lab in Canada that was able to test for COVID-19 antibodies! In my practice, being a proactive, personalized medicine physician, I felt I had to look elsewhere. I called several American labs and found one that was adding an FDA-approved antibodies platform to their offering by mid-April. I was more than happy to start helping them figure out the workflow for high-volume testing.

Around the same time, one of my clients asked me to help her manage a COVID-19 outbreak in their call center. This facility housed about a thousand people but now had about a quarter of their staff on-site to operate essential services, including suicide hotlines and financial services. Within days we went from a few cases to eight cases. They closed the facility for cleaning, but even then, Public Health requested its closure. The final count reached 32 before the call center was reopened 2 weeks later. While this may seem like any other COVID story, what was not discussed by public health officials was the information we could gather from the floor plan of the 40,000-square-foot facility.

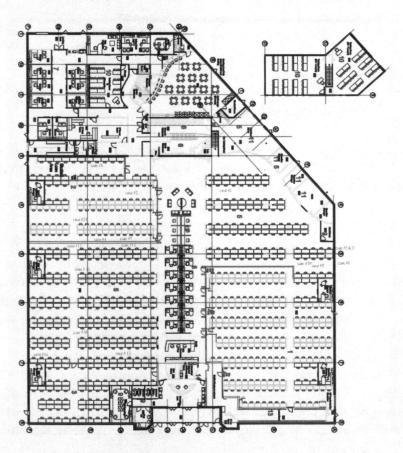

Those who tested positive for COVID-19 worked in different places all over the facility. The virus, therefore, is airborne, as social distancing did not stop the spread.

By May 2020, less than 2 months since the pandemic was announced, I was sitting on three data points that no one was talking about:

1. At least 40% of people, if not more, were asymptomatic carriers of COVID.
2. Some Canadians were likely infected outside of Canada in late 2019, early 2020.
3. The virus is airborne.

These game-changing realities meant that the public health guidelines outlining to stay away from each other and use hand sanitizer would not be adequate to control the spread. Everyone needed to wear masks, especially indoors. High-efficiency particulate air (HEPA) filters should be installed in all indoor workplaces, schools, and homes.

In the meantime, government officials assured the public that 6 feet (2 meters) was a safe distance and outlined that masks were optional, for the public, throughout the summer.

My Experience with Post-Traumatic Stress Disorder

I was glued to the news. I had to be on top of the changes going on around the world and generally stay current. The updates were fast and furious.

For the early weeks of the pandemic, I watched statistics, images, and stories that were mind-numbing and unbelievable.

• Exponential infections and death rates around the world
• Hospital staff working with inadequate PPE and begging and crying for masks, gloves, and gowns
• Emails from University Health Network, our largest hospital system in Canada, outlined how all staff could store, reuse, and re-sanitize the rationed number of masks per day

- Stories of nurses posting on YouTube to show others how to make masks from T-shirts, and gowns from garbage bags
- Coffins piled high, row on row, in Italian churches
- Refrigeration trucks acting as morgues outside New York City hospitals
- The construction of "field" hospitals in major cities
- Community stores going out of business
- Busy and long lines at food banks

Soon after an anxious week getting my son safely home from Chicago in mid-March, I lost it one night.

While watching the evening newscast of yet another horrible day for hospital doctors and nurses trying to do their best work to save lives, working with the equipment they had on hand, I began to cry.

My son said to me, "What's wrong with you? You don't need to cry. It's not you and not your patients."

That sent me off on a full-on tirade, with tears streaming down my face. I said something like this:

> It could have been me. It could be my clinic patients or my nursing home patients. While you are safely home playing video games and eating home-cooked meals and enjoying clean laundry, your dad's and mom's friends are risking their lives every day to deal with stupid people who refuse to listen to science-based health advice – to stay away from each other and simply wear a mask! They could die and leave their kids without parents.

The flood of my current fears and the anxiety I experienced during SARS came to the forefront, and I proceeded to tell him what we had had to do in 2003 to keep him safe. None of us knew who would get SARS – his parents, uncle, or grandfather, who were all working frontline SARS in Toronto.

My meltdown probably lasted 15 minutes, and I know I was sobbing and screaming at him. Needless to say, he didn't utter a word more and has never again asked me, "What's wrong?" Because *everything was really wrong.*

For many weeks during March and April, I slept just 4 hours per night. I was trying to get the masks transported to Canada, write weekly blogs to my patients, build an e-commerce site to offer antibodies testing, and fundraise for my medical school. Although I was tired by midnight, I woke up fully refreshed by 4 a.m. and worked like that for 10 to 12 weeks. I stopped exercising, as I had no gym to go to. And I snacked all day. I had palpitations again, which I often get when I am stressed out. In my dreams, I ran from bed to bed in a hospital, set up a mobile hospital, and checked in on sick medical residents in hotel rooms.

> In retrospect, I was hypomanic and certainly overstressed. I felt a need to do my part, yet I was a bystander, no longer a helpful hospital staff member in the trenches. I felt guilty in the safety of my home. I overcompensated and overworked.

Some good came out of my overdrive. To give back and not feel like I was contributing little to nothing to my colleagues in the hospital, I started a new initiative called the Masking Together Campaign. By mid-April and after just 2 weeks, this campaign raised just under $200,000 to fund PPE purchases, safe housing for quarantined medical students (residents) in hotels, and urgent research for the Faculty of Medicine at the University of Toronto to find a vaccine.

My Son Robert's Story in the Early Months of the Pandemic

I knew something was up, but I didn't think too much of it in January. Around that time, I had read a couple of articles about the virus in China and had learned about it through my project management class, where we talked about how project managers need to see all possible scenarios and plan for things.

My professor, Dr. Mark Werwath, was the first person to make me more aware of the novel coronavirus. He shared with us the fact that a hospital was built in 2 weeks and the significance of preparation and precision, something that didn't pan out too well in the United States. I was also shown a COVID-tracking dashboard created and maintained by Johns Hopkins University. The intense amount of detail and military precision baffled me and gave me some hints about the efforts taken to track something that seems impossible to control.

On January 24, Chicago announced that a female passenger had passed through O'Hare International Airport, making her the first confirmed case of COVID-19 in my town.

My mom showed up on January 30, a Thursday, prior to my birthday. I was just getting into the swing of things at the start of a new quarter at school. I typically look forward to the thought of a nice home-cooked meal in my college apartment, my home away from home.

When my mom came and settled into my apartment, she pulled me into my bedroom and opened her suitcase. In it were masks, hand sanitizers, Lysol wipes, gloves, face shields, and more supplements. Mom sat me down and started walking me through the different kinds of masks. I learned that masks had different ratings, the difference between an N95 and a surgical mask, the procedure for using commonly touched things (wearing gloves or wiping it down), and more. I got the lecture about how I needed to eat well, take my supplements, and sleep – all of which I had heard before and which sounded just like friendly Mom advice. She kept emphasizing how the PPE was like gold, but I never would have imagined any of that stuff becoming so scarce, and I blew it off.

In preparation for what she made out to be doomsday, she did a Costco run and bought food that I could seemingly live off of for the next 6 months. I continued to live normally for the next couple of months, celebrating my birthday at a bar, going out to eat with friends, and so on. But there was something still stuck in the back of my brain. I was constantly sanitizing my hands, not touching doors, and I even stopped going to the gym.

Fast-forward a couple of weeks. Things seemed to be getting a little more serious, with deaths being tallied around the world. I was under the assumption that because the United States and Canada are more developed countries, there was absolutely nothing to worry about. Something like this had never consumed these countries and I thought we would have the necessary precautions in place to protect citizens. I also thought the virus was going to be like the swine flu, or something else that couldn't spread so fast. One thing kept going through my mind: *There have to be precautions in place to contain these people, and everything will be fine, right?* Another thing that kept going through my head: *Well, if it did spread, how would I react?*

I am a bit of germaphobe, with two parents and family members who are health professionals, so I started to take the situation a little more seriously. I began telling my friends about the virus, educating them about how China built full hospitals in a couple of days and how serious the virus was. They all blew me off: "It will never come here." "Stop being paranoid!" My roommate and I even started playing this game called *Plague Inc.* – a game where the goal is to infect the entire world – as it was trending on the app store. The irony and foreshadowing of this was uncanny. Soon, I didn't touch the handlebars on the bus anymore, or any doors in my apartment building. I started wiping down the computers in the computer lab; my project mates thought I was crazy.

By the end of February, the people in my building, most of whom were from Asia (I lived in an apartment with a large concentration of international students), were all wearing masks. This was about the time that there was a COVID case at the university, and people were freaking out but also joking about the people in hazmat suits who were taking away kids on campus.

I thought to myself: *This is all coming together.* I soon knew that life was about to change very quickly. One of my friends received a shipment of N95 masks from their parents, and then a week later, the pandemic hit. By early March, Mom gave me the go-ahead to share my PPE with my inner circle of friends, providing them with the masks and shields they needed to get on a plane and go home. Campus was shutting down. And a new way of life began.

The Summer of 2020

As the COVID-19 pandemic hummed along from spring into summer, there seemed to be some hope for humanity. Trump announced an initiative that was as bold as Kennedy's desire to land an American on the moon.

"Using the resources of the federal government and the U.S. private sector, Operation Warp Speed (OWS) will accelerate the testing, supply, development, and distribution of safe and effective vaccines, therapeutics, and diagnostics to counter COVID-19 by January 2021."[21]

— *U.S. Department of Defense*

And there was another global movement afoot. On May 25, George Floyd died from asphyxiation under the knee of a police officer in Minneapolis. What followed was weeks of protests and, yes, riots – not only in the United States but also around the world. The Black Lives Matter movement exploded.

As a physician, I was torn by the worry of large gatherings, though outside. Still, I celebrated the uprising of a generation of people of all genders, race, religious beliefs – all with one cause – to bring attention to the inequalities of societies. They called out those who were privileged and naïve about the people who suffered in silence from racial inequalities and prejudice. It was heartwarming to see so many people fundamentally believing in a cause and being able to demonstrate that things need to change – all against the backdrop of hopelessness and death from COVID-19.

The movement triggered conversations we didn't want to talk about. But we did so because it was the right time and the right thing to do. As you will read in Chapter 2, racial and health injustices have always plagued our society, but they were less visible until the pandemic rooted them out. The invisible became visible. For the medical community, it was a chance for us to shine a light on healthcare disparities and the lack of access to preventive healthcare experienced by many vulnerable communities. COVID-19 research studies revealed that those with preexisting conditions, such as heart disease, diabetes, and hypertension, have a higher mortality rate than those who are otherwise healthy, but those in low-income ethnic minorities have an even higher mortality rate.

By midsummer, I was pleased to see that cases in some countries had plateaued, including Canada and Germany. The United States case counts, however, remained high, and they did in other parts of Europe.

The Beginning of Wave 2

As the overall number of cases rose around the world, one thing became certain. Everyone had an opinion as to whether the COVID-19 pandemic was a hoax or not.

It became clear that a second wave could extend into the summer and fall and would be primarily determined by:

- Personal behaviors
- Political philosophy

People decided if they would wear a mask, whether outdoors or indoors, and how much they would mingle and travel. Not all decisions were based on the science available at the time.

Politicians struggled to decide what balance to strike between the value of a human's life and the value of small businesses, when to enforce lockdowns and when to open up the economy.

And government bodies and politicians bantered back and forth trying to come up with a cohesive and logical way to roll out the vaccines.

My patients and corporate clients asked me if we would experience a second wave at the end of the summer. The summer seemed so calm. I said to them, "Absolutely!"

Here's why:

- Based on sero-surveys (testing for antibodies), the overall population infection rate around the world was still low (ranging from 1% in a Colorado town[22] to 15% in a German town[23]), but we were nowhere near the "herd immunity" needed at 75% without a vaccine.
- People continued to socialize and move between districts, trying to normalize their lives.
- Many people did not abide by public health recommendations to wear masks "whenever possible" (mask-wearing soon became mandated by fall – but it was too late).
- There was no action taken to approve more types of rapid COVID-19 detection testing (in Canada).
- The acquisition of materials and the hiring of qualified staff to

perform more PCR (polymerase chain reaction; genetics-based) COVID-19 testing was not ramped up enough to keep up with pandemic demands.

- The Canadian COVID-19 Alert app was a failure.
- Contact tracing was not sufficiently embraced anywhere in North America – electronically or by people.
- And the president of the United States did little to encourage Americans to follow safety measures throughout the summer and onward, leading to skyrocketing infection dates and deaths.

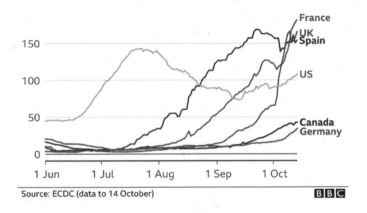

Source: ECDC (data to 14 October)

As summer progressed, the virus quietly expanded from institutional cases (mainly in hospitals, nursing homes, and workplaces) to community cases from home to home. I assumed we would start seeing higher cases for much of the northern part of North America in October, about 1 month after school, colleges, universities, and offices let people back indoors to gather.

Unfortunately, we didn't even make it to October.

Case counts started to rise sharply in Europe by late August, and in early September, the northern United States and Quebec, Canada, began experiencing their surges of COVID-19 cases.

Things changed rapidly by the fall of 2020. In the U.K., the first few cases of a new variant called 1.1.7 were identified in mid-September.[24]

It caught hold quickly, and Prime Minister Boris Johnson told the world that this variant was more contagious and likely more deadly than the first one. Parts of the U.K. sunk into another lockdown, stretching from October to early December.

In the meantime, Brazil President Jair Bolsonaro was following Trump's rhetoric and denying scientific evidence, and Brazil's case counts continued to rise throughout the late summer and well into 2021. Brazil's variant, known as P.1, also appeared to be more contagious and deadly, and a higher percentage of younger adults were falling ill with this strain than with the first one. Before the P.1 strain, the death rate of adults ages 20 to 29 was four in 10,000, but this rate increased more than threefold after P.1, to 13 in 1,000. For middle-aged adults, their death rates doubled that of their younger counterparts.[25]

The P.1 variant includes three mutations of the spike proteins. Because the vaccine partially works by detecting the virus by its spike proteins, the vaccine may have a harder time identifying this variant in the body. This can lead to more infections, deaths, and widespread transmission.

The First COVID-19 Vaccinations

By Christmas, the variant strains of the virus had spread to communities around the world. The vaccines were now the only hope, which began rolling out in amazing record time in December. In England, a grandmother received an Oxford/AstraZeneca shot on December 8. The U.K. government hoped to vaccinate four million people with a first shot before the end of 2020.[24] However, the U.K. administered only 1,380,430 by January 3,[25] so they missed the goal by quite a bit.

In the United States, a retired nurse received her first dose of a Pfizer-BioNTech vaccine on December 14.[26]

Note: Both a natural infection of SARS-CoV-2 and a vaccination against SARS-CoV-2 produce a polyclonal response of antibodies. In other words, our body produces various types of antibodies that target different parts of the spike proteins. The CDC believed that the SARS-CoV-2 virus would need to undergo multiple mutations in their spike proteins to evade the immunity induced by a vaccine or by natural infection.[27] Therefore, for now, it would appear that the vaccines would work against variant strains. Only time would tell.

The Beginning of Wave 3

By late January 2021, after the uptick of cases following the holidays, my patients and corporate clients again asked me if we would experience a third wave (despite my view that we never really got out of Wave 2). I answered, "Absolutely, but it will be worse."

Here's why:

- As people continued to travel and mingle during the summer and fall, the virus was able to spread within communities – not just within health institutions and workplaces.
- In Canada, rapid testing kits were not deployed to high-risk areas, such as nursing homes, factories, warehouses, and even schools, despite the government's stockpile of kits.[30]
- The U.K. variant arrived in Canada by January, detected in – and then spread throughout – a rural nursing home north of Toronto.[31]
- As the United States rolled out their vaccines to its citizens, Canadians waited for their supply to arrive.
- Despite the slow vaccine rollout in Canada, coupled with the infiltration of variants in the winter of 2021, provincial governments were reluctant to increase levels of lockdown measures until April 2021.

Different Experiences in Different Countries

Canada ranked around 50th in population vaccination rates during the first quarter of 2021.[32] It had no domestic supplies and was reliant on global inventory, which had proven slow to arrive. By April, the most populous provinces were well into their third wave, with high variant

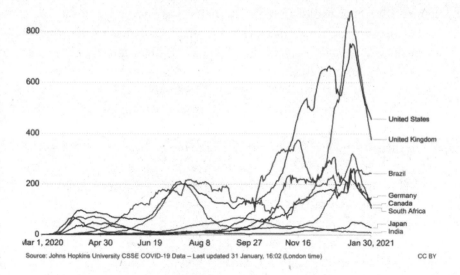

Source: Johns Hopkins University CSSE COVID-19 Data – Last updated 31 January, 16:02 (London time)   CC BY

Variant Counts - April 8, 2021		
Variant	USA	Canada
B.1.1.7 (U.K)	16,275	15,499
B.1.351 (South Africa)	386	338
P.1 (Brazil)	356	1,104

Sources: CDC and Health Canada

counts. British Columbia struggled with a high P.1 variant count, and Ontario with a high B.1.1.7 variant count.

It was apparent that most countries had not stamped out the virus from their communities. Many people defied public health guidelines and continued to flame these viral variant ambers by traveling, mingling with no masks, and generally returning to socializing within their families and friend groups. It seemed inevitable, seeing as most people have become burned out by all the rules, restrictions, and lockdowns. It wouldn't be long before things became far worse again.

The United States had a brief downturn of cases in the early fall, but by the end of 2020, cases began to rise again. The United States named it Wave 3, though many experts felt they never got out of Wave 2. Against this backdrop, vaccines rolled out rapidly across the country in early 2021. Recently elected President Joe Biden achieved his goal of 100 million vaccines administered in his first 100 days in office. In fact, he achieved his goal within his first 58 days in office. His next goal is to have 60% of Americans fully vaccinated by July 4, 2021. It appears that he will be on track.

In the race against the variants, it remains to be seen if Wave 4 will occur in the United States, Canada, and Europe in 2021 or beyond. What we know is, people have no more tolerance for lockdowns. There is no returning back to draconian public health measures.

Countries will open up by fall 2021. It's now the individual's responsibility, and perhaps businesses too, to take appropriate actions for their health and safety.

CHAPTER 2

Profile of a Pandemic Survivor

We have all struggled with the fact that the whole world has changed. Nothing will truly be the same ever again. When the pandemic first hit, all of us were in shock. All our work and home routines abruptly changed, affecting how we eat, exercise, shop, sleep, and engage with others.

As human beings, our biology thrives on routine and stability. In fact, we have a biological clock in every cell of our body. And when these clocks are thrown off course with sudden changes in how we carry out our days, our body becomes confused. We feel confused too.

Yet most of us live a shift-like lifestyle without even realizing it – especially when we have a family and a social life on weekends. Far too many of us start work on Monday mornings feeling like we need a vacation from our weekend of activities! By day, we take the kids to their team sport games, lessons, and birthday parties, and by night, we party as adults who still behave like college kids, eating and drinking too much and getting to bed late. We burn the candle at both ends. College students, pregnant women, emergency and essential workers, and business travelers are all officially classified as shift workers because they often sleep at irregular hours and sometimes without a routine.

I know that the pandemic changed my biological clock literally overnight. It suddenly impacted every minute of my waking and sleeping existence, and I experienced these changes during both the SARS and COVID-19 pandemics. I've survived, but certainly not thrived.

Researchers like American Dr. Satchin Panda point out that anything that disrupts your normal sleep–wake cycle will interfere with your circadian (day–night) rhythm. According to Panda, your eating habits and exercise routines will also impact your circadian rhythm. A weak circadian rhythm can lead to neurological, metabolic, digestive, immune, and cardiovascular diseases.[33] As you'll learn, these are all preexisting health conditions that increase your likelihood for a more severe course of COVID-19.

Thankfully, some of us found ways to improve our lifestyle and create new healthier habits during the pandemic; others had to forego their wellness routines.

> Once you are out of your lockdown, complete an audit to see how well you've adapted biologically. If you've not fared so well, let's create an action plan to correct it!

Socially, there have been more losses than gains. All sorts of rituals and gatherings, like graduations, weddings, baby showers, and funerals, were halted. Births and deaths in hospitals were eerily altered. It's been difficult to share our emotions and support each other, in celebration and in grief. Even the Queen of England, Elizabeth II, sat alone during the funeral service of her husband, Prince Philip, the Duke of Edinburgh, in April 2021.

We are social beings, and this pandemic – with all its restrictions – has made us realize how much we treasure our freedom to travel and visit with one another. This is how we, as homo sapiens, thrive and nurture one another, by being around each other.

The road to recovery from this pandemic may not be so easy to navigate, physically, emotionally, and spiritually, but I'm here to encourage you. This book will help you develop a sense of personal control again. Let's regain power over your health destiny, even if it wasn't there prior to the lockdowns. Certainly, life will be different after the pandemic. Let's put our health and well-being at the top of this list of changes. While the pandemic has created havoc, it has also forced us to rediscover ourselves. By creating new sustainable routines together, we can improve our physical and mental resiliency, anchored by deliberate self-care.

Our lives have been broken open. Let's find new opportunities for positive change.

Are You a Pandemic Survivor?

All of us have some degree of grit, but the reality is: we all experience COVID fatigue. We can't keep our guard up every day, all the time. Some of us have languished while others have stayed resilient. Nevertheless, we have all been physically and emotionally impacted.

One thing is for sure: you are a COVID-19 pandemic survivor!

INFOGRAPHIC/SURVEY – PROFILE OF A PANDEMIC SURVIVOR

[DO A SCALE 1-15] Score: add total x 2 = /100

Have you experienced?:

• Patterns of binging on junk foods
• Disrupted exercise routine
• Increased use of recreational drugs – including alcohol and cannabis
• More feelings of stress, anxiety, and sadness
• Disturbed sleep with COVID-19-related dreams
• An increased workload from your job and homelife
• Reduced work travel and commuting
• Sense of social isolation
• Friction with spouse/partner and children at home
• Financial strains due to change in employment

If you scored high on this questionnaire, you are not alone.

How each of us responds to stress (and especially during this lengthy COVID-19 pandemic) depends on several variables, such as:

• Background (for example, spiritual, cultural, and educational experiences)

- Social support network of family and friends
- Financial situation
- Health and emotional background
- The community you live in

Let me share with you some recent research data related to the first wave of the pandemic. I don't think it will surprise you, but these numbers may comfort you by acknowledging that you are human and "normal" during unprecedented times.

Are You in This Demographic?

According to the Centers for Disease Control and Prevention (CDC) in Washington D.C., those who may be more significantly impacted by stress include people who:

- Are at higher risk for severe illness from COVID-19 (older people; people of any age with certain underlying medical conditions, such as obesity, heart disease, diabetes, hypertension, and autoimmune diseases)
- Are a parent of a child or teen
- Care for family members and loved ones
- Are frontline workers, such as healthcare providers and first responders
- Are essential workers who work in the food industry
- Have existing mental health conditions
- Use substances or have a substance use disorder
- Have lost their jobs, had their work hours reduced, or experienced other major changes to their employment
- Have disabilities or developmental delays
- Are socially isolated from others, including people who live alone and people in rural and frontier areas
- Belong to certain racial and ethnic minority groups
- Do not have access to information in their primary language
- Are experiencing homelessness
- Live in congregate (group) settings

Health Issues

Obesity

The COVID-19 pandemic has caused many of us to struggle with our weight, and the patients in my practice are no exception, as evidenced by the annual health assessments we performed in the second half of 2020. My patients, on average, gained a "few pounds." They ate and drank more, including alcohol, and their active lifestyles dramatically changed to shelter-in-place existences – if not shelter-in-chair zooming for 8-plus hours a day. Snacking on comfort foods became a norm for months, and it didn't help that many started to do more home baking!

And for those who already had weight issues, a common challenge faced by approximately half the population of North America, they found that the struggle to keep the weight under control was real.

Obesity Numbers

A study published by the UT Southwestern Medical Center Weight Wellness Program in Clinical Obesity found that among their patients during COVID-19[34]:

Often, health issues – which includes weight challenges – are exacerbated by financial circumstances. Of those 123 people in this study:

- 10% lost their jobs.
- 20% said they could not afford a balanced meal.

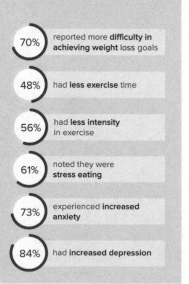

70% reported more **difficulty in achieving weight** loss goals

48% had **less exercise** time

56% had **less intensity** in exercise

61% noted they were **stress eating**

73% experienced **increased anxiety**

84% had **increased depression**

We know that those who are obese (those who have a body mass index, or BMI, of over 30) often have comorbidities such as heart disease and diabetes. Therefore, the complication of weight gain appears to have a greater impact than just putting on a few pounds. For many it can become a tipping point for the onset of obesity-related medical conditions and even contracting (and dying from) COVID-19.

Overall, most of my patients saw an increase in their insulin levels, which is a sign of increased insulin resistance, a risk factor for developing diabetes despite having normal blood sugar control numbers. (See Chapter 2 to learn more about these biomarkers.)

Mental Illness

Beyond weight-control issues that impact our physical health, these lockdowns have also significantly affected our mental well-being. The pandemic has shone a light on the fragility of those with a tendency to develop mental illness and a lack of sufficient services to address a growing need.

Two general-population polls done in 2020 by Angus Reid Institute[35] and Morneau Shepell[36] found that 81% of Canadian workers felt the pandemic had negatively impacted their mental health.

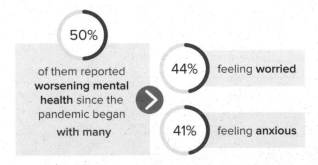

50% of them reported **worsening mental health** since the pandemic began **with many**

44% feeling **worried**

41% feeling **anxious**

There are health associations between the experience of quarantine and symptoms of anxiety and post-traumatic stress, sometimes with long-term effects. This not only impacts adults but also their children too. Kids who quarantine with their parents experience post-traumatic stress scores that are four times higher than children who do not quarantine.[37]

However, people with existing serious mental illnesses are at the greatest risk.

Those who suffer from schizophrenia are more likely to contract COVID-19 and experience worse health outcomes compared to the general population.[38] This is due to the nature of their mental illness, underlying physical health problems caused by compromised diets, drug abuse, sleep disorders, and poor social determinants of health.

ALCOHOL AND CANNABIS USE AND ABUSE

Substance abuse from alcohol and drug consumption, as well as overdoses, have certainly been pervasive within many communities in the past. But these have been on the rise since the pandemic hit. Across Canada, those with severe substance abuse issues were unable to easily access harm-reduction sites, resulting in a significantly higher number of deaths due to overdose since the beginning of COVID-19. The British Columbia Coroners Office reported that the overdose death toll in September 2020 was more than double the 60 fatalities recorded in the same month in 2019.[39]

The United States 2020 nationwide data on overdose deaths will not be available until late 2021. Researchers predict it may jump upwards by at least 27% compared to pre-pandemic levels. If this prediction becomes a reality, it will be the largest single-year percentage increase in the past 2 decades.[40]

Although 70% of Canadians reported their alcohol consumption had stayed the same since the pandemic began, 18% reported drinking more and 12% reported drinking less because they lacked the social opportunities to do so.

Binge drinking, or heavy episodic drinking, remained a concern well into the fall of 2020 as the second wave of lockdowns began. Because alcohol is an addictive drug, binging can often lead to many health problems, such as alcohol abuse. The longer a person engages in this coping strategy, the harder it is to stop the dependency.[41]

BINGE DRINKING DEFINED: On average, men consume five or more drinks, and women consume four or more drinks, in approximately 2 hours. (CDC)

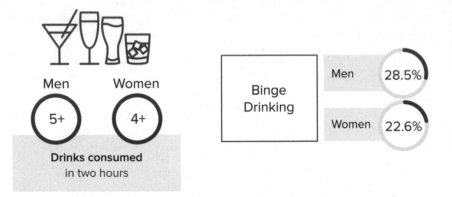

Men   Women

5+   4+

Drinks consumed
in two hours

Binge Drinking

Men   28.5%

Women 22.6%

Not all age groups reported the same increase in their drinking habits. Those under 55 years of age consumed more alcohol than other older age groups. The younger population between age 18 and 34 reported that both their consumption of alcohol and cannabis had increased.

The reasons most cited for the increase in consumption were:

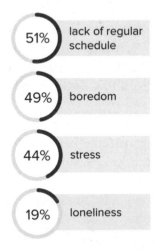

51% lack of regular schedule

49% boredom

44% stress

19% loneliness

Women were more likely to cite stress (57%) as a reason for consuming more alcohol (compared to men, 32%), while men were more likely to cite boredom (54%) as a reason for the increase (compared to women, 44%).

STATISTICS AT A GLANCE

Increased use of alcohol by age:

- Canadians 55-plus years of age (10%) ages 35 to 54 (25%) and 18 to 34 (21%).

Increased use of cannabis by age:

- 18 to 34 years of age had increased (14%) compared to those 35 to 54 (6%) and 55-plus (1%).[42]

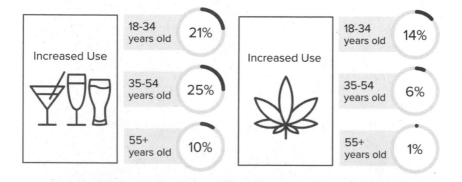

The following questions concern information about your potential involvement with drugs <u>not including alcoholic beverages</u> during the past 12 months. Carefully read each statement and decide if your answer is "Yes" or "No." Then, circle the appropriate response beside the question.

In the statements, "drug abuse" refers to (1) the use of prescribed or over the counter drugs in excess of the directions and (2) any nonmedical use of drugs. The various classes of drugs may include: cannabis (e.g., marijuana, hash), solvents, tranquilizers (e.g., Valium), barbiturates, cocaine, stimulants (e.g., speed), hallucinogens (e.g., LSD), or narcotics (e.g., heroin). Remember that the questions do not include alcoholic beverages.

Please answer every question. If you have difficulty with a statement, then choose the response that is mostly right.

These questions refer to the past 12 months.

Answer with Yes or No

1. Have you used drugs other than those required for medical reasons?
2. Have you abused prescription drugs?
3. Do you abuse more than one drug at a time?
4. Can you get through the week without using drugs?
5. Are you always able to stop using drugs when you want to?
6. Have you had "blackouts" or "flashbacks" as a result of drug use?
7. Do you ever feel bad or guilty about your drug use?
8. Does your spouse (or parents) ever complain about your involvement with drugs?
9. Has drug abuse created problems between you and your spouse or your parents?
10. Have you lost friends because of your use of drugs?
11. Have you neglected your family because of your use of drugs?
12. Have you been in trouble at work because of drug abuse?
13. Have you lost a job because of drug abuse?
14. Have you gotten into fights when under the influence of drugs?
15. Have you engaged in illegal activities in order to obtain drugs?
16. Have you been arrested for possession of illegal drugs?
17. Have you ever experienced withdrawal symptoms (felt sick) when you stopped taking drugs?
18. Have you had medical problems as a result of your drug use (e.g., memory loss, hepatitis, convulsions, bleeding, etc.)?
19. Have you gone to anyone for help for a drug problem?
20. Have you been involved in a treatment program specifically related to drug use?

Scoring:

A factor analysis of the 20 items has indicated that the DAST is essentially a unidimensional scale. Accordingly, it is planned to yield only one total or summary score ranging from 0 to 20, which is computed by summing all items that are endorsed in the direction of increased drug problems. Only two items are keyed for a "No" response: "Can you get through the week without using drugs?" and "Are you always able to stop using drugs when you want to?" A DAST score of six or above is suggested for case-finding purposes, since most of the clients in the normative sample score six or greater. It is also suggested that a score of 16 or greater be considered to indicate a very severe abuse or a dependency condition.

We realize that good mental health is important to the well-being of all our communities. Prior to the pandemic, mental health services were always in high demand. Post COVID-19 pandemic, even more people will seek emotional support and counseling.

Impact on Communities

Almost a year into the COVID-19 crisis, a global McKinsey survey done among employees showed that a diverse group of people are having the hardest time, both in their workplaces and with balancing work and homelife. They include working parents, women, LGBTQ+ employees, and people of color.[43]

And despite companies trying to support their employees during this pandemic, challenges remain.

Families

At the beginning of this chapter, I referenced Dr. Panda's research about our biological clocks. We have a biorhythm. It's prefaced on our lifestyle routines. Our bodies and minds thrive on predictable schedules. This all changed in a matter of weeks in March 2020.

What usually took years to transform, happened in just days. Daycares and schools closed, and classrooms moved to online learning. Parents either worked from home or were laid off. If you didn't have internet access at home or own enough devices, everyone in the household became technology-compromised. In fact, 15% of families surveyed in Ontario, Canada, didn't have access to the internet at home when school went virtual.

Workplaces changed overnight too. Our in-person collaborations with colleagues became endless days of video conferences, and inter-actions with our customers had to be reinvented. Some organizations were already cloud-based, had e-commerce platforms, and were far more able to pivot with their team. If your company was not ready for remote working, it became a 24–7 job to get it there, with kids beside you "going to school."

Everyone struggled globally in every way.[44]

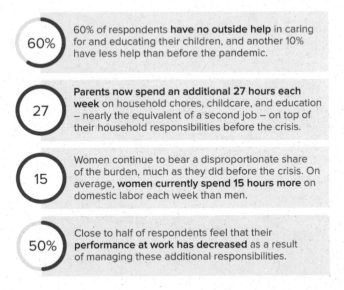

60% — 60% of respondents **have no outside help** in caring for and educating their children, and another 10% have less help than before the pandemic.

27 — **Parents now spend an additional 27 hours each week** on household chores, childcare, and education – nearly the equivalent of a second job – on top of their household responsibilities before the crisis.

15 — Women continue to bear a disproportionate share of the burden, much as they did before the crisis. On average, **women currently spend 15 hours more** on domestic labor each week than men.

50% — Close to half of respondents feel that their **performance at work has decreased** as a result of managing these additional responsibilities.

Stress at work and home skyrocketed.

There was simply nowhere to hide and take respite. One study showed that parents with children under 18 living in the home were more likely to feel depressed (29.1%) compared to adults without children (18.9%). In fact, 57% of caregivers met the criteria for depression.[45, 46]

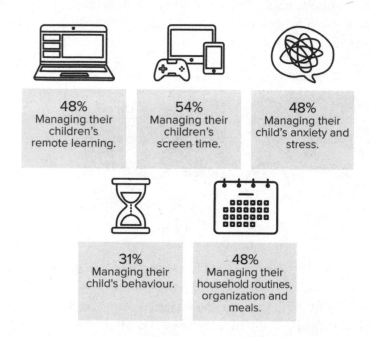

48% Managing their children's remote learning.	**54%** Managing their children's screen time.	**48%** Managing their child's anxiety and stress.
31% Managing their child's behaviour.	**48%** Managing their household routines, organization and meals.	

It became "game on" day and night. For many, it was playing out as well in our dreams while we slept! (See Chapter 9 to learn more about sleep.) Thankfully, people became resourceful, and many companies, friends, neighbors, and extended family members pitched in to transform each other's lives to "make it work."

But some families had to make lose-lose decisions. They couldn't find the help they needed to take care of their children, and their job – deemed essential – meant they had to be at work. Without help, Mom, who usually has the lower-paying job, often had to stay behind to take care of the children at home, giving up her career.

Women

Many women have socially accepted that they do more; they have two jobs, one at a workplace and one at home. There is data to support that a woman's workload has increased during this pandemic. Women now spend approximately an additional 15 hours a week more on domestic labor than men. And women with children at home are now adding an extra 4 to 6 hours a day to care for them. This impact on women is happening regardless of income.[47, 48]

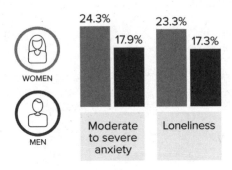

Undoubtedly, the pandemic will have a long-term negative impact on the gains made by women that improve gender diversity in the workplace. Unfortunately, the losses have started. Women, especially women of color, are more likely to have been laid off during this pandemic. More than one in four women are contemplating "downshifting" their careers or leaving the workforce completely.[49] The risk to corporations losing women in leadership and future women leaders is real and must be addressed by organizations globally.

> The workplace and homelife have transformed forever. As we come out of lockdown and recover from COVID-19, employers must do more to alleviate the new pressures on families and, in particular, on women.

Domestic Abuse

As noted earlier, families are struggling, and when we are under pressure, we sometimes "lose it." We don't need statistics to tell us that. Spouses argue with one another and with their children. In one study, many admitted they were tougher on their kids when they were stressed.[50]

We're likely all guilty in some way with our emotions during the lock-downs. And in some cases, unfortunately, arguments escalate into more serious verbal or physical conflict at home.

While domestic violence can happen to both genders, one in four women experience intimate partner violence (IPV) compared to one in 10 men. Such violence can be physical, emotional, sexual, or psychological. People of all races, cultures, genders, sexual orientations, socioeconomic classes, and religions are susceptible to experiencing IPV.[51]

During the early stages of the pandemic, stay-at-home orders created a dangerous situation for some. It left many victims trapped with their abusers. Domestic-violence hotlines prepared for an increase in demand, but many organizations experienced up to a 50% drop in the number of calls they received.[52] Experts know that rates of IPV had not decreased. It became clear that victims were unable to safely connect with their services.

Nellie's Shelter

In mid-April (2020), a young pregnant woman living at Nellie's went for a routine prenatal appointment. As a precaution, her doctor tested her for COVID-19 even though she had no symptoms.

It came back positive.

Nellie's staff quickly helped her move into one of the city's quarantine centers to protect shelter residents and staff. But soon after, other women and their children started to show symptoms of the virus.

To date there have been 11 confirmed cases in the shelter. The good news is that no one has needed to

be hospitalized and everyone is recovering well.

In a shelter with 40 beds that was originally only designed for 16, it's challenging to practice physical distancing. There simply isn't enough space. It's the reality of shelter living, especially in an old shelter.

To halt the COVID-19 outbreak, all of the women and their children moved out of the shelter and into a nearby hotel. Nellie's is not the first shelter to have to do this. Staff moved to the hotel as well to continue to create positive spaces for the women through our programs and workshops that offer therapeutic healing, personal growth and distraction during this challenging and stressful time.

It's a complete shift in how we do business right now. COVID-19 is impacting our bottom line.

We're still here and we'll still be here at the end of this. When women who are at home and need us, we're still going to be here for them when they call.

Excerpted from Nellie's Shelter newsletter, with permission.

Masking Together Challenge #2 is a proud donor to Nellie's Shelter in Toronto, Canada.

Nellie's Shelter is supported by our Masking Together Challenge and received 2,000 masks, 60 face shields, 140 bottles of hand sanitizer, and COVID-19 cleaning materials – all approved by Health Canada.

Violence against children is another kind of abuse that exists in our society. During this pandemic, traditional watchdogs, such as other family members, teachers, childcare providers, and healthcare clinicians, have had less contact with children. This has created fewer opportunities to assess, recognize, and report signs of child abuse. Experts believe the decrease in the reporting of suspected abuse during the lockdowns reflects a lack of screening rather than a decrease in actual abuse.[53] [54]

Eventually the data will reveal the true degree of increased domestic violence during this pandemic. But the women's shelters across the nation will tell you that the need for safe housing has never been greater.

Homelessness

The needs of shelters in North America have increased in general, as more people become homeless for the first time because of economic hardships. Although shelters stay open, they have had to reduce the number of beds because of the need to social distance. In cities with hotels, these spaces are being transformed to support the many people who are socially marginalized, including abused women and their children. But it's a temporary fix if the economy doesn't recover quickly and people can't find reemployment.

> "It's a shame it took something like COVID for people to see that people need a home and that we're all the same."[55]
> — *Raquel Winslow, person living with homelessness from nearby* Port Coquitlam, *interviewed on CBC*

Charities do receive some government funding, and they are also accepting donations from donors. They receive some medical-grade PPE too, but the amount they receive runs out quickly or just barely suffices (these PPE supplies are also offered to clients who drop in to their community center).

The need is great within our vulnerable communities. As a society, we need to also protect our invisible frontline healthcare workers, those who support the most vulnerable people living in homeless encampments and in shelters. They are often lost in the conversation, compared to the frontline staff working in hospitals and nursing homes that have specialized public relations staff and budgets to amplify their stories of need.

Pandemics within the Pandemic

The COVID pandemic has revealed the income gap inequalities within various communities of our societies. The impact has disproportionally hit those deemed to be vulnerable, often defined as those who live in crowded or communal housing or even shelters and are generally less healthy and don't have the time or means to practice wellness. Populations who are deemed to be at higher risk of contracting COVID-19 and dying from it include racialized peoples (especially Black/African American and Hispanic/Latino persons and Indigenous communities[56]), people with disabilities, people with dementia, new immigrants, refugees, and workers in low-wage or precarious employment.[57]

In one study in Scotland, the impact of socioeconomic status on 30-day mortality in hospitalized patients with COVID-19 infection was far greater in people termed "more deprived."[58]

The coronavirus *does* discriminate.

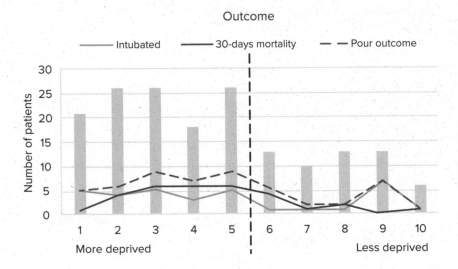

Outcome

Similar findings have been noted in other countries. For example, in England, the Office for National Statistics has shown, using an index of multiple deprivation, that the rate of deaths related to coronavirus was as much as 88% higher in most deprived areas compared with the least deprived areas.[59]

> We are not safe as a society until all our communities become safe and rid of COVID-19, first by stopping its spread by using masks and vaccinations, and then by addressing the social injustices that COVID-19 has revealed to each of us.

Frontline Workers Meeting Coronavirus Head-On

For most of this chapter, we've focused on those who have had to quarantine and isolate. But not everyone has been so lucky. Some people had to confront the COVID-19 virus every day they went to work.

I can't begin to express enough thanks to our essential frontline workers; they not only keep us safe, but also save lives, feed us, and get us to where we need to go every day. While we have honored them with food, song, and gifts, we can't forget about them when they "return home" from this invisible war against this virus. Only when they have a moment to reflect on how they stared death in the face for this past year and more will they feel the full impact of their sacrifice.

Essential Workers

People who provide a range of essential services during the pandemic are at an increased risk of severe mental health difficulties. From the post-SARS era, studies found healthcare workers continued to experience post-traumatic stress disorder and other mental illnesses for up to 3 years after the end of the SARS pandemic.[60]

Governments, hospitals, nursing homes, and even grocery chains were not providing all their frontline workers with essential PPE during the first wave of the COVID-19 pandemic. This impacted their mental health negatively. Healthcare providers (including, but not limited to, physicians, nurses, personal support workers, social workers, and occupational therapists) became particularly more vulnerable due to their greater risk of exposure to the virus, concerns about infecting loved ones, and their risk of dying.[61]

Their fears were and are legitimate. At the peak of the 2020 summer wave of the pandemic, frontline healthcare workers who had adequate PPE were still three times more at risk of COVID-19 infection than the general public.[62]

Healthcare workers who contracted COVID-19 and survived are far more likely to develop a mental illness in the longer term, based on studies done of healthcare workers who contracted SARS while on the job (compared to non-healthcare workers).[63] [64]

Those who provided direct COVID-19 patient care, those who had a friend or family member who became infected, and those who have been quarantined may be two to three times more likely to develop symptoms of post-traumatic stress than those not exposed to these conditions.[65]

In China, one study found that 40% of their physicians and nurses who provided care to COVID-19 patients were experiencing depression, anxiety, insomnia, and/or distress.[66]

Post-pandemic, how we fund mental health resources both in the public and private sectors will determine if we can all recover fully from the pandemic experience.

Oprah Winfrey Quotations[67]

"The whole point of being alive is to evolve into the complete person you were intended to be."

"So go ahead. Fall down. The world looks different from the ground."

"Challenges are gifts that force us to search for a new center of gravity. Don't fight them. Just find a new way to stand."

In the next section of this book, let's focus on you. How well have you survived the pandemic of the century? How well have you coped, or has it taken a toll on your physical and mental health?

Next steps: measuring the impact on you, a survivor of the COVID-19 pandemic.

ASSESSING THE TOLL

CHAPTER 3

Know Your Numbers

The year 2020 changed the way we live, work, socialize, exercise, and think about the world we live in. To begin our health assessment journey to move forward and thrive, let us start with something we can all relate to, and rely on, the gold standard for basic physical biomarkers: our vital signs. While it may seem boring and basic, our heart rate, blood pressure, weight, body mass index, respiratory rate, and blood oxygen levels all give us information about how well our critical organs are functioning.

A very rudimentary portion of our brain, the brain stem, takes care of these vital life functions without us even trying.

Heart Beats and Wave Pressure

The medulla portion of our brain stem transfers neural messages to and from the brain and spinal cord. The sympathetic and parasympathetic branches of our autonomic system are comprised of a complex network of nerve fibers and cells that secret chemicals to stimulate muscle contractions of the heart. If our heart beats regularly within a certain range during rest and exercise, we consider the heart to be functioning well.

Our heart rate is the number of times our heart pumps to push blood around the body per minute. The heart rhythm is a pattern of heart beats. An arrhythmia is an abnormal heart rhythm, which many people may experience over their lifetime.

Arrhythmias are caused by an abnormality in that electrical conduction system, which can be triggered by a number of factors, such as genetics, coronary heart disease or heart valve disease, medications, supplements, and stimulants (such as coffee, alcohol, cannabis, and stress). While we often attribute irregular rhythms to fast-beating heart rates, an arrhythmia can also be slower. Some arrhythmias are more serious

How to Measure Your Heart Rate by Taking Your Pulse

Every heartbeat creates a wave of pressure as blood flows through your blood vessels. Your wrist is a good place to feel the pressure wave, or your pulse. Certainly, you might have a watch that measures not only your heart rate but also your rhythm. But to do it the old-fashioned way, you'll need a clock or watch that measures seconds.

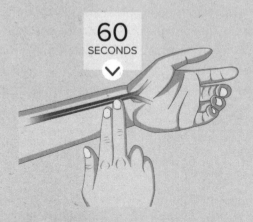

1. Hold one of your hands out with your palm facing up.
2. Place the first and middle fingertips of your other hand on the inside of your wrist at the base of your thumb.
3. Press lightly and move your fingers around until you feel your pulse.
4. Count how many beats you can feel in 60 seconds.
5. You can also feel the rhythm of your pulse and check if it's regular or irregular.[68]

than others. Those who notice their arrhythmia often feel anxious, even if their condition is not harmful. However, for others, it can impact their quality of life, causing shortness of breath, chest pain, and even loss of consciousness due to insufficient oxygen circulating around the body.

Some people may say they are experiencing "palpitations," which feels like a fluttering or their heart is pounding. Others describe palpitations as feeling like a thud or movement in their chest or up their neck, or through their ear when they are lying down.

Most people who get these sensations usually don't have a serious heart condition, but palpitations can feel unpleasant and may cause distress. They are common, and especially when experiencing a lot of stress and anxiety, with adrenaline pumping and overstimulating the heart. If you're concerned about palpitations, see your physician. They may order an electrocardiogram to see how the electrical impulses are firing and to evaluate the heartbeat and rhythm.

Ectopic beats are early or extra heartbeats that can cause palpitations, and they can make it feel like your heart has skipped or missed beats. Most people have ectopic beats at some time in their lifetime; generally, these are nothing to worry about – unless you feel symptoms of shortness of breath or chest pain.

Blood Pressure

Your blood pressure is another important physical biomarker of your heart health. If you have high blood pressure or hypertension, your heart will be working hard to push blood forward, and the high force of the blood flow can harm your arteries and cause organ damage, especially your heart, kidneys, brain, and eyes. Poorly controlled high blood pressure can raise the risk of heart attack, heart failure, stroke, kidney disease, and blindness.[69]

There are two numbers to record when determining your blood pressure. The top number, called the systolic number, measures the pressure caused by your heart's contraction as it pushes blood through your blood vessels. The bottom number is your diastolic pressure and measures the pressure in your arteries when your heart relaxes between beats. While a diagnosis of high blood pressure may be worrisome, unusually low blood pressure can also cause health issues, as there is not enough blood circulation around your body.

Which number is more important?

Generally, more attention is given to systolic blood pressure numbers. It is a well-accepted major risk factor for cardiovascular disease for people over 50. In most people, systolic blood pressure rises with age because of the increasing stiffness of large arteries caused by a long-term buildup of plaque, leading to increased cardiac and vascular disease incidence. Far too often, it is related to a sedentary lifestyle, bad eating habits, and poor sleep.

The risk of death from ischemic (low oxygen) heart disease and stroke doubles with every 20 mm Hg systolic or 10 mm Hg diastolic increase among people between the ages of 40 and 89.[70]

Cumulative Incidence of Cardiovascular Events in Women (Panel A) and Men (Panel B)

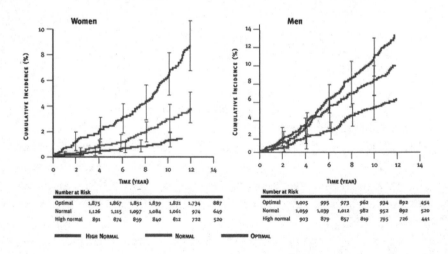

Understanding Blood Pressure Readings

What do your blood pressure numbers mean?

The only way to know if you have high blood pressure or hypertension is to take your blood pressure.

BLOOD PRESSURE CATEGORY	SYSTOLIC mm Hg (upper number)		DIASTOLIC mm Hg (lower number)
＞ Normal	< 120	and	< 80
＞ Elevated	120 - 129	and	< 80
＞ High Blood Pressure (Hypertension) Stage 1	130 - 139	or	80 - 89
＞ High Blood Pressure (Hypertension) Stage 2	140 +	or	90 +
＞ Hypertensive Crisis (consult doctor immdiately)	180 +	and/or	120 +

Source: American Heart Association.

Note: The abbreviation mm Hg means millimeters of mercury. Mercury was used in the first accurate pressure gauges and is still used in medicine today as the standard unit of measurement for pressure.

A normal blood pressure of less than 120/80 mm Hg is considered within the normal range. If your results fall into this category, continue with your heart-healthy habits.

Elevated blood pressure is defined as readings that consistently range from 120 to 129 systolic and less than 80 mm Hg diastolic. People with elevated blood pressure are likely to develop high blood pressure, and, therefore, steps need to be taken to manage this at-risk condition.

Hypertension Stage 1 is defined as blood pressure that consistently ranges from 130 to 139 systolic or 80 to 89 mm Hg diastolic. Your physician will prescribe lifestyle changes and may add blood pressure medication to your routine based on your atherosclerotic (plaque formation) cardiovascular disease risk factors.

Hypertension Stage 2 is defined as blood pressure that consistently ranges at higher than 140 systolic and 90 mm Hg. With this blood pressure, you will likely need a combination of blood pressure medication and lifestyle changes.

A hypertensive crisis requires immediate medical attention if your blood pressure readings suddenly exceed 180 systolic and 120 mm Hg. Wait 5 minutes and retest your blood pressure. If your readings are still high, contact your healthcare practitioner immediately.[71]

Overall, the prevalence of hypertension among North American adults is around 30%, according to the Centers for Disease Control and Prevention (CDC). High Blood pressure increases dramatically with age.[72]

High blood pressure can be caused by many factors, including genetics (such as ethnicity) and gender. The prevalence of hypertension increases with age, from 7.5% among adults ages 18 to 39, to 33.2% among adults ages 40 to 59, to 63.1% among adults age 60 and over. After 65, women are more likely than men to develop high blood pressure. Pregnancy, birth control, and menopause (all life-cycle hormone changes) can increase the risk of developing high blood pressure.[73, 74, 75]

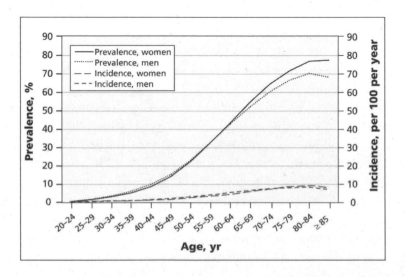

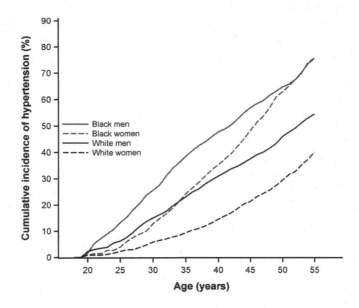

Other factors increase your risk of developing hypertension and are cumulative over our lifetime, such as diet (especially with high salt intake), lack of cardiovascular exercise, and smoking. The good news is, high blood pressure can be lowered through lifestyle changes to reduce your risk.

What Is the DASH Diet?

There are few diets that I would recommend everyone adopt, but the Dietary Approaches to Stop Hypertension (DASH) diet is one of them because it is reasonable and improves blood pressure and hence overall cardiovascular health. While we think of the heart as a major beneficiary of low blood pressure, the brain will also benefit from this diet, reducing your risk of stroke and related diseases affecting the blood vessels, such as dementia.[76, 77]

The DASH diet was developed to lower blood pressure without medication. The research was sponsored by the National Institutes of Health (NIH) in the United States. The DASH diet can be viewed as a lifelong approach to healthy eating and is in line with dietary recommendations to prevent osteoporosis, cancer, heart disease, stroke, and diabetes.

Amazingly, this diet can lower your blood pressure in as little as 2 weeks. Over time, your systolic blood pressure could drop by 8 to 14 points, which can make a significant difference in your overall vascular health risks.[78]

	Food	Daily Servings
	Vegetables & Fruits 1 SERVING: 1/2 cup (or 1 cup greens) or 1 piece fruit	11
	Grains 1 SERVING: 1/2 cup pasta or rice or cereal or slice bread	4
	Low-fat Dairy 1 SERVING: 1 cup milk or yogurt or 1½ oz. cheese	2
	Legumes & Nuts 1 SERVING: ½ cup beans or ¼ cup nuts or 4 oz. tofu	2
	Poultry, Fish & Lean Meat 1 SERVING: ¼ lb. cooked	1
	Oils & Fats 1 SERVING: 1 Tbs.	2
	Desserts & Sweets 1 SERVING: 1 tsp. sugar or 1 small cookie	2
	Wild Card Poultry, Fish, Lean Meat or Oils & Fats or Grains or Desserts & Sweets	1

The core premise of the DASH diet is to lower sodium intake to 2300 mg at most per day, which is equivalent to 1 teaspoon (5 mL) of salt. Ideally, intake could decrease to 1500 mg per day. Unfortunately, a typical North American diet soars at upwards of 3400 mg of sodium per day or more.

Before you blame your home cooking, you should know that most dietary sodium (over 70%) comes from packaged and prepared foods.

> Some foods that don't taste salty can still be high in sodium; therefore, using taste alone is not an accurate way to determine if a food's sodium content is high. Sodium has multiple uses – it's important in curing meat, baking, thickening, retaining moisture, and enhancing flavor, and it's also a preservative. Common food additives – including monosodium glutamate (MSG), sodium bicarbonate (baking soda), sodium nitrite, and sodium benzoate – all contain sodium and contribute to the total amount of sodium listed on the Nutrition Facts label (in the United States) and the Nutrition Facts tables (in Canada).[79]

The Relationship Between Sodium and Blood Pressure

Sodium, or salt, attracts water, and a diet high in sodium draws water into the bloodstream. This can increase the volume of blood and subsequently your blood pressure. Because blood pressure generally rises as you get older, limiting your sodium intake becomes even more important as you age.

10 Easy Tips for Reducing Sodium Consumption

1. **Read the Nutrition Facts label.** Eat less than 100% daily value (DV; less than 2300 mg) of sodium each day.
2. **Prepare your own food when you can.** Limit packaged sauces, mixes, and "instant" products.
3. **Add flavor without adding sodium.** Try a no-salt seasoning blend of herbs and spices instead of salt or MSG.

4. **Buy fresh food only or fresh frozen whole foods (fruits and vegetables).** Choose only fresh meat, chicken, and seafood (rather than processed and prepared foods, which often include salt water or saline).

5. **Watch your veggies.** Buy fresh or frozen and canned vegetables with no salt added.

6. **Give it a rinse.** Wash sodium-containing canned foods with water, whenever possible.

7. **Choose low-sodium.** Opt for no-salt-added nuts and seeds, and avoid snack products (such as chips and pretzels). Better still, try carrot and celery sticks instead.

8. **Reduce your condiments.** The sodium in condiments can add up. Choose light or reduced-sodium condiments, add oil and vinegar to salads, and use only a small portion of seasoning from flavoring packets.

9. **Reduce your portion size.** Less food equals less sodium. Consume a smaller plate of food, especially when eating out.

10. **Make lower-sodium choices on menus.** Ask the chef to prepare your meal without salt and request sauces and salad dressings on the side, and use less of them.

Source: FDA – Sodium in Your Diet Use the
Nutrition Facts Label and Reduce Your Intake[80]

How to Measure Your Own Blood Pressure

You may have heard of white coat syndrome, and nowhere is it more prevalent than when patients get their blood pressure taken at their health practitioner's office. When a person is anxious about their blood pressure reading in front of a health professional, the adrenaline starts to flow, which temporarily increases heart rate and blood pressure. Therefore, regularly measuring your own blood pressure can help you determine if your blood pressure is, in fact, high.

HOW TO TAKE ACCURATE BP READINGS
- Buy an automatic blood pressure cuff (it works with just the press of a button), rather than a hand-pumped one.

- Take your blood pressure first thing in the morning (before doing any activities) and at the end of your workday, at about the same time every day.
- Use the same arm each time.
- Remove clothing from your arm completely.
- Sit quietly with your feet flat and your back resting against the back of a chair for at least 5 minutes before beginning and during measurement.
- Wrap the cuff snugly around your upper arm (two fingers should fit between the blood pressure cuff and your arm). The edge of the cuff must be 1 inch (3 cm) above your elbow.
- Rest your arm comfortably on a table or another firm surface. The cuff should be at the level of your heart.

TIPS FOR A MORE ACCURATE READING
- Do not measure your blood pressure when you are upset or in pain.
- Do not smoke tobacco or drink caffeine (found in coffee, tea, colas, and some sports drinks) for 30 minutes beforehand.
- Do not talk or watch TV during the test.
- Take one reading and record your blood pressure. (When you first use the cuff, you may be nervous, so don't worry the first few times if they're a bit high.)[81]

Breathing

"Inhale the present, exhale the past and the future."[82]
— *Leticia Rae, social media influencer and aspiring personal development coach*

Breathing is the process of moving air in and out of your lungs to extract oxygen from your environment and exhale carbon dioxide gas from your body. This interaction requires a thin membrane in your lungs to transfer these gases back and forth from your bloodstream. Like your heart, this process is controlled by the medulla in your brain, which controls blood flow to and from your lungs and other organs.

We never think about it, but it takes many muscles to move air in and out of our lungs. The lungs themselves don't have muscle but are often described as air-filled sponges. They rely on other muscles to draw air into the lungs. Muscles in your chest and abdomen contract to create a slight vacuum around your lungs. This "sucks" air in. When you exhale, the muscles relax and the lungs deflate on their own.

Your breathing muscles include the:

- Diaphragm
- Intercostal muscles (the muscles between the ribs)
- Abdominal muscles
- Muscles of the face, mouth, and pharynx
- Muscles in the neck and collarbone area

Source: NIH[83]

Respiration Rate

The respiration rate is the number of breaths you take in a minute and is usually measured while you're at rest. You can measure your respiration rate by counting the number of times your chest rises. When a doctor observes your respirations, they may also note whether you have any difficulty breathing.

A normal respiration rate for a healthy adult at rest ranges from 12 to 16 breaths per minute.

BLOOD OXYGEN SATURATION

Oxygen saturation is defined as the amount of oxygen that's in your arteries as a result of the gas exchange and circulation system of your lungs and heart. To function properly, your body requires an oxygen saturation between 95% to 100%. Anyone with an oxygen saturation level below 90% will require medical attention and, likely, supplemental oxygen.

There are two ways of measuring oxygen saturation: an arterial blood gas (ABG) test and a pulse oximeter. ABGs are performed only by doctors in a hospital setting for patients who are critically ill. The more common pulse oximeter is used elsewhere, such as in ambulatory settings and homes.

There are many reasons why our breathing rate and oxygen saturation might change. Those of us who have traveled to higher elevations, such as when we go downhill skiing, may have noticed this phenomenon. Higher elevation environments have a lower oxygen concentration, so our breathing and, therefore, our oxygen saturation drop. Over time our body adjusts, and then breathing becomes more comfortable.

However, medical conditions, acute or chronic, are the most common reasons for low blood oxygen levels, such as asthma, chronic obstructive lung disease, emphysema, and interstitial lung damage. These can be caused by infections or environmental exposure to toxins, such as cigarette smoke, pollution, asbestos, or caustic chemical vapors.

Obesity is another factor and can lead to apnea (a sudden stop in breathing), especially during sleep. More people than ever are getting tested in sleep clinics, and doctors have discovered that apnea happens to far more people than we previously thought.

In 2019, a group of researchers reviewed the literature for reliable prevalence data for obstructive sleep apnea in 16 countries. They estimated that 936 million men and women ages 30 to 69 years have mild to severe obstructive sleep apnea. The number of affected individuals was highest in China, followed by the United States, Brazil, and India.[84]

COVID-19 Pneumonia

Respirologists have noticed that many patients with COVID-19 experience low blood oxygen levels just days before seeking medical attention because of shortness of breath. These specialists believe that a pulse oximeter can be lifesaving, as it can serve as an early warning signal that a patient may be developing viral pneumonia.[85]

> Pneumonia is a respiratory infection where the lungs' air sacs, called alveoli, are filled with fluid or pus, causing them to collapse and oxygen levels to drop. Patients can develop chest pain and significant breathing problems.

Thanks to the Internet of Things, pulse oximeters, such as the Circul Ring, are now being widely used to detect low oxygen due to respiratory distress. Many of these types of devices also measure both heart rate and blood oxygen saturation.

COVID-19 patients can be sick for a week or so with fever, cough, upset stomach, and fatigue, but they often go to the ER only when they become short of breath. By then, often their pneumonia has been developing for days, so by the time they are short of breath, they are already in critical condition. Many patients do not report any sensation of breathing problems even though their chest X-rays show diffuse pneumonia and their oxygen saturation is below normal.

> Normal oxygen saturation for most people is 95% to 100%; COVID-19 pneumonia patients can experience oxygen saturations as low as 50%.

Respirologists now recognize that COVID-19 pneumonia initially causes a form of oxygen deprivation called silent hypoxia. It is "silent" because of its insidious, hard-to-detect nature.

WHAT IS SILENT HYPOXIA?

In hypoxia, oxygen saturation in the body is insufficient. Because oxygen is vital for the energy production in cells (cell respiration), insufficient oxygen supply causes cell damage. Some tissues in the body are more sensitive to hypoxia than others. The brain is particularly sensitive – an acute lack of oxygen causes brain cells to die after just a few minutes, which quickly leads to irreparable brain damage.

Usually, hypoxia is noticeable quite quickly. The skin can turn bluish (cyanosis), and people can also experience headaches, palpitations, shortness of breath, and dizziness.

Unfortunately, this is not the case with silent hypoxia. Although the oxygen saturation of those affected drops sharply, they do not experience any of the symptoms mentioned.

Richard Levitan, an emergency physician in Littleton, New Hampshire, commented in *The New York Times*: "I realized that we are not detecting the deadly pneumonia the virus causes early enough and that we could be doing more to keep patients off ventilators – and alive. . . . It's like nothing I've ever seen before."[86]

While tools such as a Circul Ring do not replace an actual COVID-19 test, they can serve as another alert for the early detection of a COVID-19 infection. The Circul Ring can help identify patients who have silent pneumonia sooner and alert them to seek medical attention.

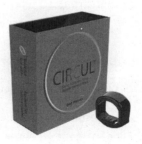

Anybody who has tested positive for the coronavirus should have pulse oximetry monitoring for 2 weeks, the period during which COVID-19 pneumonia typically develops.

Anyone with cough, fatigue, and fevers should also have pulse oximeter monitoring – even if they have not tested for the virus and even if their swab test was negative (tests are not 100% accurate).

Body Weight and BMI

People die from COVID-19 because of the virus's inflammatory impacts. When inflammation happens because of an infection in our lungs, we call it pneumonia. And when it attacks our vascular system, it can lead to a heart attack and stroke.

I was not surprised, therefore, when I learned that COVID-19 primarily impacts those with preexisting conditions, including obesity.[87]

Recent research shows that COVID-19 patients with obesity had a higher mortality rate compared to those without obesity. These obese patients also demonstrated more severe negative change in their lungs and had higher levels of lymphocytes, triglycerides, interleukin 6 (IL-6), C-reactive protein (CRP), cystatin C, alanine aminotransferase (ALT), and erythrocyte sedimentation rate (ESR) – which all greatly influence disease progression and the likelihood of a poor prognosis of COVID-19.[88]

Obesity

Obesity has been by far the most serious public health concern of the modern industrialized world. The epidemic rise in obesity and diabetes means we are rapidly aging prematurely as a society. Children are diagnosed with diabetes at a younger age. Most alarming, so many children are now expected to die before their parents: not because of war or infection, but from complications of diabetes – beginning with cardiovascular disease and heart attack.

Many people don't realize that obesity still significantly increases their risk of at least 18 chronic diseases. Some of these can be fatal. The three big killers – heart disease and stroke, diabetes, and cancer – top the list, followed by other conditions like high blood pressure, arthritis, and liver and gall bladder disease.

If you have visceral (abdominal) fat outside your body, it means there's fat on the inside of your body as well – specifically in your organs too, which impairs their function.

Definition: Body Mass Index

BMI is a measure of your body fat based on height and weight. The BMI categories are:

- Underweight = less than 18.5
- Normal weight = 18.5–24.9
- Overweight = 25.0–29.9
- Obese = 30.0–34.9
- Morbidly obese = 35.0 and greater

To calculate BMI, we use the equation of mass (kg) ÷ height (m)^2. For example, a man who weighs 210 pounds (95 kg) and is 5 foot 10 inches (1.778 m) in height would be calculated as $95 \div 1.778^2$, which equals a BMI of 30, or obese.

Having heathy physical biomarkers assumes that our heart and lungs are functioning well. But it does not offer us insights about the looming risks of developing chronic medical conditions, especially conditions that lead to the top three killers.

Recurring rounds of COVID lockdowns and changes to our work, school, and home routines created social isolation and changes to our lifestyles. Ultimately, COVID-19 has affected our physical and mental health whether we were infected or not. Our health behaviors changed to cope with the situation. Most of us gravitated to comfort lifestyles, altering our diets, exercise routines, and sleeping habits.

But did these behavioral changes impact your biochemical biomark-ers? These biomarkers can determine if you have increased your risks to many lifestyle-modifiable health issues, including cardiovascular dis-ease, diabetes, arthritis, and even sleep apnea.

Let's explore some essential biochemical biomarkers to determine how well your body's organs are functioning now.

CHAPTER 4

Is Your Body Functioning Well?

How well have you been coping with the pandemic? With your lifestyle completely altered – whether you are a frontline worker or switched to working from home or became unemployed with children in the house – nothing is the way it used to be.

Once lockdown restrictions were put in place, many of us realized how much our lifestyles revolved around visiting friends and even family for entertainment. We looked forward to our movie nights and restaurant meals. Sunday brunch had offered us a special event to plan and look forward to. After COVID-19 hit, many of us had to learn how to cook and bake! And we did it with our families and children over Zoom. Although comfort foods took center stage for a few of those early months, many later tried to find ways to eat better at home – takeout was not a long-term solution.

Most gyms closed, and at first, this allowed us to stop working out with a trainer, if we'd had the luxury to do so before. We paused the routine of going to a spin bike, yoga, or fitness class. But soon we didn't feel so well, sitting in front of our computers and eating. We gained weight, and our backs began to hurt. We got cabin fever. Gradually we found new ways to exercise, just in time for the spring season. Like the birds, we got busy in nature. We walked and ran. And as fall settled in, we discovered that online training videos and virtual sessions were a reasonable and convenient option so long as we could motivate ourselves to do it. Gym equipment supplies flew off the shelves and became out of stock online as many, including me, realized we just needed a Plan B.

Our sleep patterns also changed, partly because of what we ate, drank, and the intensity of our new workdays – now working from home and pivoting to virtual collaborations, all with kids underfoot and helping them with online school. Some of us slept better because we cut back on the caffeine and alcohol. But for others, the disrupted and restless sleep crept in. The stressors we brought to bed stayed with us all night.

> Our lifestyle choices alter our metabolic functions. How and what we eat, the types of exercises we do, and the quantity and quality of our sleep change our chemical and hormonal markers.

Let's review the most common biochemical and hormonal markers impacted by our lifestyles in this chapter. These markers, in turn, impact our risk for diseases such as heart disease, stroke, diabetes, and cancer. Such preexisting conditions impact your ability to fight off other diseases, including COVID-19. It's best to be proactive and begin now to see if you are at risk for them. To assess your current overall health, visit your healthcare professional and submit your lab work as soon as possible.

Assess Your Risks for Metabolic Dysfunction and Inflammation

This set of biochemical markers flags your risk for developing cardiovascular disease and diabetes. Obesity is a major cause of driving metabolic illness.

Know the Biomarkers of Glycation and Diabetes

Glycation occurs when cross-links (a crisscrossing) of proteins develop at the cellular level. This can cause your organs and DNA to function poorly.

This process directly affects your gene expression and protein production. Glycation is caused by poorly controlled glucose levels in our bloodstream, poor diet, insulin surges, and insulin receptor insensitivity. You might recognize these medical words in definitions for diabetes, prediabetes, and insulin resistance.

Biomarkers that can measure glycation are made up of many diabetes risk markers. These include the commonly tested fasting blood sugar glucose level. Although constantly high blood glucose levels define that you have diabetes, I believe that taking such snapshots in time can't really determine if you're developing diabetes because this marker becomes elevated only when your body systems are broken and you can no longer cope with the sugar load. Sadly, by then, it's too late! Using a car tire analogy, why wait until all the air is out of the tire to do something about it? Once there is a hole in a tire, it is defective forever. The same is true with the diagnosis of diabetes. Once you have diabetes, you always have diabetes. At best, you will perhaps be a diabetic who is in "good control" of your high blood glucose levels through diet and medications.

I believe that hemoglobin A1C (HgbA1c) is a more effective biomarker than a fasting blood sugar measurement. I've been using this marker as a guide to show my patients they're starting to show the signs of diabetes with abnormal HgbA1c levels.

It measures the 3-month control of your blood sugar levels in your body. In this test, we measure the degree of sugar coating on your hemoglobin (red blood cell), which swims in your body for a 3-month life span. Both the American and Canadian Diabetes Associations advocate using HgbA1c as the better standard to diagnose diabetes.

Other high-potential tests to measure your diabetes risk include measuring your insulin level. This hormone is critical in regulating blood sugar levels. Certainly, this biomarker can predict insulin resistance, a condition where a person's cells have difficulty responding to the normal actions of the insulin hormone.

Researchers have shown a relationship between insulin resistance and diabetes. There is no one test for insulin resistance, but having high blood sugar, triglycerides, and LDL ("bad") cholesterol, plus low HDL ("good") cholesterol, is a likely sign you are developing insulin resistance. IR is especially strong when it coincides with an increase in your body mass index (BMI).[89]

Insulin

This hormone is most commonly associated with diabetes. It is secreted from your pancreas in response to how many carbohydrates you eat. Its sole goal is to keep your body's blood sugar stable – not too high (diabetes) or too low (hypoglycemia).

The classical form of diabetes is known as type 1, which is caused when the pancreas can't produce insulin, leading to very serious complications of significantly high blood sugar levels. The lifesaving treatment is insulin injections.

What few people realize is that most people diagnosed with diabetes today have type 2 diabetes. This form of diabetes is not initially caused by the body's inability to produce insulin (type 1), but rather the body's inability to use the insulin being produced because of obesity – insulin resistance. Your body produces a great deal of insulin to cope with the rising blood sugar levels, and then the pancreas tires and stops producing insulin. At that point, these diabetics require insulin injections. As their insulin resistance develops, a lot of damage is done inside the body. When insulin resistance increases, oxidative stress also rises, causing more cellular damage.

Oxidative Stress

Oxidation, or oxidative stress, is the amount of damage inside and outside of cells created by free radicals. Free radicals are a natural by-product of your body's physiological processes (burning oxygen to create energy for the functioning of cells). They can also enter your body through the environment – from pollution, smog, cigarette smoke, and radiation from sunlight.

One way to really "see" oxidative stress at work is to watch what happens to a fresh apple after it's been sliced and left to "age" on your kitchen counter. The oxygen molecules in the air of your home begin to damage the exposed flesh of the fruit, browning it. But sprinkle lemon juice on the slices, and the freshness of the fruit is extended. Why? Lemon juice contains the antioxidant vitamin C, and antioxidants can stop the effects of free radicals by neutralizing the damaging chemical process.

Unfortunately, free radicals negatively affect our genetic structure and cell function by attacking our DNA and damaging cell membranes. This exposes sensitive genetic material that can become prone to mutation and destruction. This process spreads much like rust on metal. The compromised areas intensify and, in the process, weaken your body's ability to neutralize free radicals – leading to chronic diseases such as heart disease, diabetes, cancer, and arthritis, as well as age-related conditions like wrinkles and stiff joints. In other words, the more free radicals you have, the more damage done to your body.

The cellular damage caused by COVID-19 is still being researched. But it is clear that the SARS-CoV-2 virus activates the host's immune response, which results in the secretion of inflammatory factors known as cytokines. A cascade of cytokine reactions increase oxidative stress and inflammation, and this ultimately results in the death of infected cells – and potentially the death of the host.[90]

Eating and drinking antioxidants or taking them as supplements can decrease the damage done by free radicals and by oxidative stress in your body. Another way to do this is to increase the body's production of natural antioxidants, especially with other healthy lifestyle choices, such as exercising, eating a balanced diet, and minimizing your emotional stress.

Cholesterol

Today, measuring cholesterol is as common as measuring blood pressure. But it's not enough to just learn the total and estimated levels of "good" (HDL) and "bad" (LDL) cholesterol. Standard tests calculate these values. We need to go deeper. We need to study all the sub-particles of cholesterol. Certain subsets of LDL are more atherogenic (plaque building) than others, and some HDL subtypes are more helpful in reducing this risk, such as alpha-1. The level of triglycerides (a type of fat in our bloodstream) also plays an important role in understanding our risk for diabetes. An overload of blood sugar causes the liver to store the sugar as these light-chain fats.

If you have visceral (abdominal) fat outside your body, it means there's fat on the inside of your body as well – specifically in your organs too, which impairs their function. For example, people with visceral fat on their liver, or fatty liver, often have impaired cholesterol metabolism, and we know that cholesterol affects our vascular health.

Here's my analogy of how vascular plaque develops in our arteries. Imagine a smooth plastic pipe. Now pour lard through it. Will it stick? No. But what if you gouge the inside of the tube, scratching it up? Now the lard gets caught in the wall. That's what high levels of sugar are doing in your bloodstream. Sugar gouges the lining of your artery walls. Cholesterol comes along, and sticks to the wall. Add a bit of calcium, and voila! You have plaque – a permanent scab that grows and, in time, causes atherosclerosis (a hardening of the arteries) and later narrows, causing heart attacks and strokes. We know that cholesterol is a variable contributing to cardiovascular disease.

We have also learned that, in addition to diabetes, the presence of cardiovascular disease also contributes to the poor prognosis of COVID-19.[91]

Both of these chronic health conditions increase the incidence of inflammation. And ultimately it is inflammation of the arteries in our heart and lungs that leads to many causes of death in some cases of COVID-19, namely heart attack, stroke, and pulmonary embolism.[92, 93, 94]

Know the Biomarkers of Inflammation

Inflammation is a cellular response we can blame on certain proteins that damage target tissues and change both our gene expression and the formation of new proteins. What determines the rate of our tissue damage is the imbalance of good anti-inflammation and bad inflammation that is compounded inside and outside our cells. This inflammatory process is controlled by nutrients known as fatty acids, especially along the cell walls.

What does inflammation look like? Well, say you take a tumble off your bike. What do you see after grazing your skin from the fall? Initially, your skin is red and bleeding. Shortly afterward, the injured area is sticky, and then a scab forms. When the scab falls off, the skin can often be contracted, thin, and tender. How well the repair process goes will determine the level of scarring. Where there's scarring, there's tissue damage.

The effects of inflammation depend on your net balance of inflammation proteins to your anti-inflammation nutrients. Just like we have debt-to-equity ratios in the financial world, there is a commonly used ratio of inflammation to anti-inflammation that measures the acid levels in our body (arachidonic acid, which is a polyunsaturated omega-6 fatty acid, and fatty acids, specifically eicosapentaenoic acid, or EPA, an omega-3 fatty acid). There are also other proteins commonly measured to detect inflammation, such as C-reactive protein (CRP) and homocysteine. Both are considered risk factors for the development of cardiovascular damage. In particular, vitamin B_6 has been shown to reduce the inflammation of these inflammatory proteins.[95]

COVID and the Heart, Part 1

I first met my client, age 42, about a year before the pandemic. Like many of my clients, he has a successful business with more than 50 employees and countless contractors. As owner and founder, his job is to bring in the business. Before COVID, this meant that he was wining and dining prospective clients, enjoying large meals at lunch and dinner that often included red meat, wine, and even a cigar. While in his youth, he had been an elite athlete and extremely fit. But as the years passed, and given the time crunch, exercise went by the wayside. Sleep deprivation became the norm, with early starts and late nights, especially with business travel. In summary, self-care and self-discipline fell from the priorities list.

Here were his vital signs:

- BP: 131/86 Heart Rate: 71 (stage 1 hypertension)

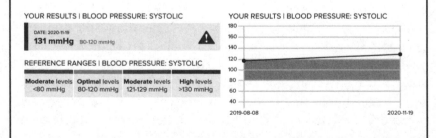

YOUR RESULTS | BLOOD PRESSURE: SYSTOLIC

DATE: 2020-11-19
131 mmHg 80-120 mmHg ⚠

REFERENCE RANGES | BLOOD PRESSURE: SYSTOLIC

Moderate levels	**Optimal** levels	**Moderate** levels	**High** levels
<80 mmHg	80-120 mmHg	121-129 mmHg	>130 mmHg

YOUR RESULTS | BLOOD PRESSURE: SYSTOLIC

(chart y-axis: 180, 160, 140, 120, 100, 80, 60, 40; x-axis: 2019-08-08 to 2020-11-19)

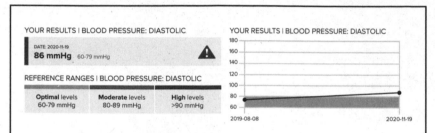

YOUR RESULTS | BLOOD PRESSURE: DIASTOLIC

DATE: 2020-11-19
86 mmHg 60-79 mmHg ⚠

REFERENCE RANGES | BLOOD PRESSURE: DIASTOLIC

Optimal levels 60-79 mmHg	Moderate levels 80-89 mmHg	High levels >90 mmHg

YOUR RESULTS | BLOOD PRESSURE: DIASTOLIC (graph: 2019-08-08 to 2020-11-19)

- BMI: 33 Weight: 231 pounds (105 kgs) (obese)

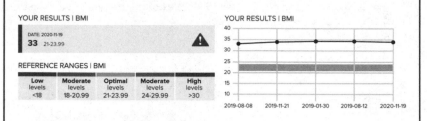

YOUR RESULTS | BMI

DATE: 2020-11-19
33 21-23.99 ⚠

REFERENCE RANGES | BMI

Low levels <18	Moderate levels 18-20.99	Optimal levels 21-23.99	Moderate levels 24-29.99	High levels >30

YOUR RESULTS | BMI (graph: 2019-08-08 to 2020-11-19)

Biochemistry:

- Cholesterol: Triglycerides: 0.8 LDL 1.92, HDL 1.38 mmol/L (these readings fall in the normal range because he takes a statin medication to lower his overall cholesterol)

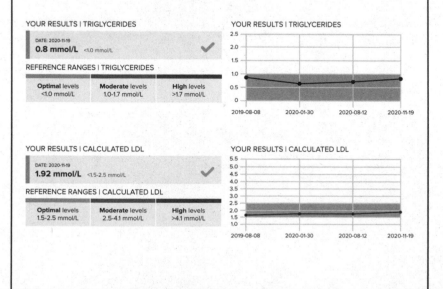

YOUR RESULTS | TRIGLYCERIDES

DATE: 2020-11-19
0.8 mmol/L <1.0 mmol/L ✓

REFERENCE RANGES | TRIGLYCERIDES

Optimal levels <1.0 mmol/L	Moderate levels 1.0-1.7 mmol/L	High levels >1.7 mmol/L

YOUR RESULTS | TRIGLYCERIDES (graph: 2019-08-08 to 2020-11-19)

YOUR RESULTS | CALCULATED LDL

DATE: 2020-11-19
1.92 mmol/L <1.5-2.5 mmol/L ✓

REFERENCE RANGES | CALCULATED LDL

Optimal levels 1.5-2.5 mmol/L	Moderate levels 2.5-4.1 mmol/L	High levels >4.1 mmol/L

YOUR RESULTS | CALCULATED LDL (graph: 2019-08-08 to 2020-11-19)

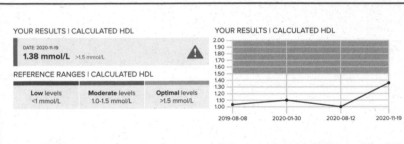

YOUR RESULTS | CALCULATED HDL

DATE: 2020-11-19
1.38 mmol/L >1.5 mmol/L

REFERENCE RANGES | CALCULATED HDL

Low levels	Moderate levels	Optimal levels
<1 mmol/L	1.0-1.5 mmol/L	>1.5 mmol/L

YOUR RESULTS | CALCULATED HDL

- **Metabolic Markers: Fasting sugar 6.9 mmol/L, A1C 5.8%, insulin 271 pmol/L (this reading demonstrates significant prediabetes due to insulin resistance)**

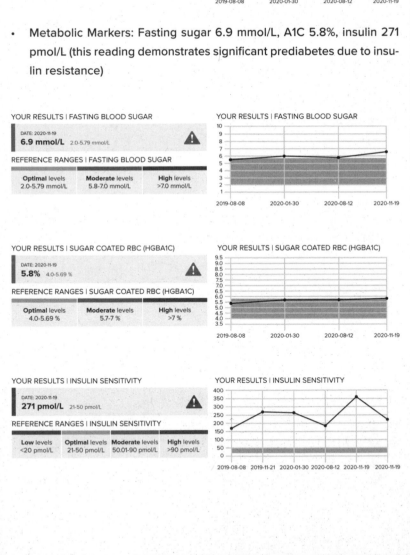

YOUR RESULTS | FASTING BLOOD SUGAR

DATE: 2020-11-19
6.9 mmol/L 2.0-5.79 mmol/L

REFERENCE RANGES | FASTING BLOOD SUGAR

Optimal levels	Moderate levels	High levels
2.0-5.79 mmol/L	5.8-7.0 mmol/L	>7.0 mmol/L

YOUR RESULTS | FASTING BLOOD SUGAR

YOUR RESULTS | SUGAR COATED RBC (HGBA1C)

DATE: 2020-11-19
5.8% 4.0-5.69 %

REFERENCE RANGES | SUGAR COATED RBC (HGBA1C)

Optimal levels	Moderate levels	High levels
4.0-5.69 %	5.7-7 %	>7 %

YOUR RESULTS | SUGAR COATED RBC (HGBA1C)

YOUR RESULTS | INSULIN SENSITIVITY

DATE: 2020-11-19
271 pmol/L 21-50 pmol/L

REFERENCE RANGES | INSULIN SENSITIVITY

Low levels	Optimal levels	Moderate levels	High levels
<20 pmol/L	21-50 pmol/L	50.01-90 pmol/L	>90 pmol/L

YOUR RESULTS | INSULIN SENSITIVITY

- CRP 1.42 (inflammation marker is higher than ideal of <1.0)

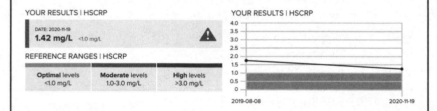

Diagnostic Imaging:

- The ultrasound showed fatty liver (meaning he was also obese on the inside).
- The CT angiogram in summer 2020 showed that two arteries were narrowed by 25%. (This is not unusual for many people over time – but ideally it should be 0%.)

During the Christmas holidays, like so many people, my patient hosted a family gathering. One person in attendance had the virus, and days later, everyone tested positive for COVID-19. My patient experienced some typical symptoms – cough, fever, chills, and aches. He was doing fine for about 2 weeks, but then he became extremely sweaty and tired, and he felt some chest pain. After 24 hours of extreme fatigue, he decided to get checked out at the hospital.

Testing at the ER showed he had had a heart attack.

Commentary

Living with prediabetes or heart disease is worrisome and challenging as is it. But if you contract COVID and have one of these conditions, you could quite literally die.

The question is: How did he have a heart attack when his major heart arteries were only 25% narrowed? Inflammation can cause a rapid increase, from 25% to 50% narrowing. And how does a 50% blockage cause a heart attack, an episode resulting from a heart muscle that is damaged from lack of oxygen? A change from 25% to 50% is equivalent to a 100% increased narrowing.

When the body is out of shape, the heart can't handle such a drastic drop in oxygen delivery; it can't adapt quickly enough. Therefore, heart muscle damage ensues. Thankfully, my patient lived through this health incident, but did it need to happen?

The virus exacerbates preexisting conditions. We need to be proactive and reduce our risks for complications in the future.

Hormones

The Role of Hormones

The word *hormone* comes from the Greek and means "to set in motion" or "to spur on," and this is exactly what our hormones do. They set in motion the many biological functions that keep us healthy. And because our biological system is designed to keep the body and mind in balance, we must keep a careful balance of the 80 different hormones that work together continuously to maintain optimal health.

Your endocrine system is responsible for balancing hormones. It's made up of glands that produce and send hormones, acting like messengers to all parts of your body. Your endocrine system regulates processes such as metabolism, cell growth, cell aging, and cell death. The target cells receive the hormone, which triggers the cell to act in a specific way – to synthesize proteins, replicate, or repair itself. All of these commands are part of your body's overall response to its environment. As well as controlling the actions of individual cells, hormones also send feedback messages to your different glands, indicating if more or less hormone is needed in your body.

The following are some of the more important metabolic and well-being hormones that I focus on in daily practice.

Growth Hormone

High blood sugar levels and high insulin levels affect other hormones. In particular, growth hormone levels drop. The pituitary gland produces human growth hormone (hGH) in our brain. Most of us are born with high levels of growth hormone. Children with genetically low growth hormone experience stunted growth, and hormone replacement is used to ensure that they can grow. In contrast, children and young adults who have too much growth hormone develop a condition called acromegaly, which many believe former president Abraham Lincoln had, as he grew to be six-foot-four (1.93 m).

As we age, our growth hormone levels drop. By the time we are in our 60s, our growth hormone level is much lower than during our 20s. But after puberty, after we've grown as tall as we're ever going to, we still need growth hormone to heal and repair our adult tissues.

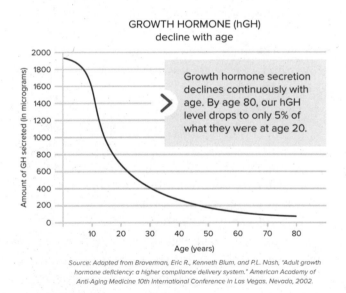

GROWTH HORMONE (hGH)
decline with age

Growth hormone secretion declines continuously with age. By age 80, our hGH level drops to only 5% of what they were at age 20.

Source: Adapted from Braverman, Eric R., Kenneth Blum, and P.L. Nash, "Adult growth hormone deficiency: a higher compliance delivery system." American Academy of Anti-Aging Medicine 10th International Conference in Las Vegas, Nevada, 2002.

As growth hormone levels drop over time, symptoms of aging increase. These include:

• Decreased energy and fatigue
• Decreased physical performance, stamina, and recovery

- Increased body fat with decreased lean muscle mass
- Decreased bone mass – rising risk for osteoporosis
- Increased LDL ("bad") cholesterol and triglycerides, lower HDL ("good") cholesterol, and higher risk of cardiovascular disease
- Weakened immune system
- Reduced metabolic rate – increased intolerance to cold temperatures
- Sleep dysfunction
- Mood alteration – anxiety, depression, and decreased libido
- Impaired memory and ability to concentrate

Although our pituitary gland releases small amounts of hGH throughout the day, most of our hGH is secreted at night, peaking 1 to 2 hours after the onset of deep, rapid-eye-movement (REM) sleep. Therefore, it's essential to get enough good sleep to ensure the optimal secretion of growth hormone every day. Strenuous exercise every day and sufficient intake of high-quality protein are also critical for optimizing your hGH secretion.

During a pandemic lockdown, when we tend to eat more carbohydrates and less protein and we exercise less, not only does hGH secretion drop, but so does our testosterone.

Testosterone

Testosterone is mostly responsible for men's sexual development during puberty, and it is critical in maintaining erectile function and libido. This hormone also declines with age. By the time a man reaches 80, testosterone levels have dropped to only 20% of what they were in his 20s.

Testosterone plays an important role in the formation of male organs and in secondary sex characteristics, such as facial and pubic hair growth, increased muscle mass, and the development of a deeper voice. This hormone is considered an anabolic, or body-building, hormone that promotes increased muscle mass in both sexes. Testosterone binds to receptors in your muscle cells. This increases the rate of nitrogen retention, which stimulates muscle growth while preventing muscle breakdown. Some experts believe that testosterone aids in weight loss because this hormone "burns" fat. Metabolically, testosterone cuts the rate of glycation by helping your body maintain lean body mass, reduce visceral fat and total cholesterol, and control your blood sugar.

Testosterone, in turn, can impact estrogen.

Estrogen

In women, there are three types of estrogens. Estrone (E1) is the predominant estrogen during menopause; estradiol (E2) is the most potent and dominant during a woman's reproductive years; and estriol (E3) is most abundant during pregnancy. All three types of estrogens are synthesized from the male sex hormone testosterone.

Estrogen is mainly a female hormone, but it is also found in small amounts in men. In women, estrogen is produced primarily in their ovaries. Each month, estrogen stimulates ovulation. It also helps prepare their uterine lining to receive a fertilized egg. Estrogen is also responsible for physical maturation, including filling out of the breasts and hips and developing the female reproductive organs during puberty. In men, this hormone is responsible for the maturation of sperm.

Metabolically, estrogen accelerates the burning of fat, increases HDL ("good") cholesterol while decreasing LDL ("bad") cholesterol, and reduces bone resorption, which boosts bone formation. It's no wonder menopausal women notice a 10% to 15% weight increase, a sudden increase in their cholesterol levels, and the development of osteoporosis (bone loss).

The Role of Nutrients

During the early days of the pandemic, I urged my patients to increase their supplement regimen to increase nutrient intake, reduce inflammation load, increase their antioxidants to reduce free-radical damage, and boost immunity. Some of my physician colleagues would advocate that eating well should be sufficient. However, in my clinic, where we measure all critical nutrients, we frequently discover less-than-ideal levels in many of my patients who rely on nutrition alone. The goal is to reduce our risks of COVID-19 complications and improve our chances for a full recovery should we contract the virus, so we should do all we can to maintain optimal health.

It's almost impossible for anyone to get enough of the right nutrients from food these days. And even if we consume enough nutrients and vitamins in our diet, many of us can't absorb the nutrients we need because of stress, allergic reactions, inactivity, or medications. What's more, as we get older, our bodies become less efficient at digesting and absorbing.

There's definitely an overlap in the function of different nutrients. For example, alpha lipoic acid and the B vitamins reduce glycation, but the B vitamins are also associated with reducing inflammation along with the omega-3 fatty acids, vitamin C, and vitamin D.

As for oxidation, alpha lipoic acid and vitamin C are powerful antioxidants. But iron can also be considered an antioxidant when used in small doses; however, it can become an oxidant in large doses. Magnesium can prevent both glycation and inflammation. The amino acids glycine, glutamine, and arginine all prevent oxidation and glycation. And arginine can boost low growth hormone levels. Immunity boosters include zinc, vitamin C, and a mushroom extract known as active hexose correlated compound (AHCC).

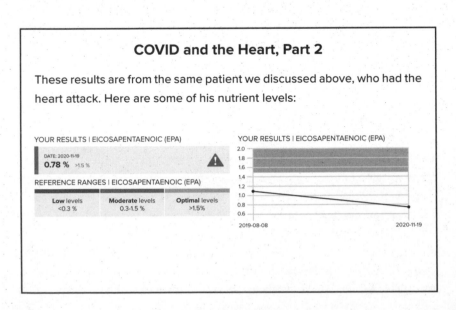

COVID and the Heart, Part 2

These results are from the same patient we discussed above, who had the heart attack. Here are some of his nutrient levels:

YOUR RESULTS | EICOSAPENTAENOIC (EPA)

DATE: 2020-11-19
0.78 % >1.5 %

REFERENCE RANGES | EICOSAPENTAENOIC (EPA)

Low levels	**Moderate** levels	**Optimal** levels
<0.3 %	0.3-1.5 %	>1.5%

YOUR RESULTS | EICOSAPENTAENOIC (EPA)

2019-08-08   2020-11-19

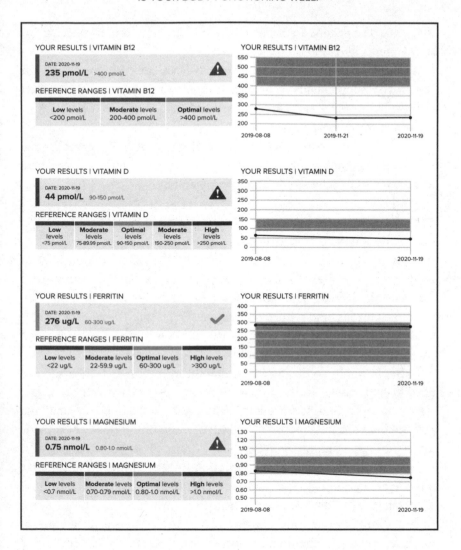

Can You Count on Supplements to Live Healthier and Longer?

There are three camps of believers when it comes to the use of supplementation. Naysayers believe that you will get enough nutrition if you just eat the right meals, and that taking supplements is a waste of money. The pro-supplement users will point to studies that suggest that taking some form of vitamins and minerals will help with our health and longevity. Then there are those in the middle ground who select a few supplements here and there, just in case.

Here's my view: supplements do have benefits. But you can't ask one or two supplements to perform miracles and be the magic bullets to prevent or treat your heart disease, diabetes, or cancer. This is asking too much of any supplement.

And, as with anything on the topic of our health, it's complicated. Some studies that initially showed promise have fallen short. Here are a few examples of the recommended supplements:

OMEGA-3 FATTY ACIDS: EICOSAPENTAENOIC ACID (EPA) AND DOCOSAHEXAENOIC ACID (DHA)

Omega-3 fatty acids are beneficial in reducing inflammation in your body. There is strong evidence that omega-3 fatty acids can improve your heart health, decrease joint inflammation, reduce the intensity and number of headaches, and reduce depressive symptoms. The only downside to omega-3 fatty acids is that they are also considered a natural blood thinner, so bruising may occur if taken in high doses.

What becomes confusing is the amount of omega-3 fatty acids you need to help counteract the inflammatory process. We know the omega-3 fatty acids from plant sources convert into ALA (alpha linolenic acid) and provide only a small amount of the EPA. Therefore, it does not provide many anti-inflammatory benefits.

Fish oil has the highest concentration of EPA. However, not all fish oils are created equal. The common daily dose of a fish oil capsule is 1000 mg, but this does not mean you will absorb 1000 mg of EPA. Some capsules will liberate only 250 mg of EPA and others will liberate as much as 600 mg. A therapeutic dose is between 2000 and 4000 mg of EPA.

When purchasing an omega-3 fish oil, go for the blended oils – salmon, sardines, anchovies, and mackerel. Be wary of just salmon oil (due to the high mercury content). Also, pure cod liver oil will have a higher concentration of vitamin A, increasing the risk of lung cancer in smokers.

B VITAMINS

The B vitamins are essential for metabolism because they transform our proteins, fats, and carbohydrates into energy. They play a role in our nervous system health, supporting our hormone function and blood cell formation. You need them to maintain energy during periods of chronic stress and help support the adrenal glands, which secrete cortisol – your stress-response hormone.

Vitamin B_6, B_{12}, and folic acid prevent inflammation in blood vessels by reducing the protein homocysteine. Vitamin B_6 is central in enhancing many neurotransmitter pathways as well. These include serotonin (your "happy hormone" pathway), epinephrine, and norepinephrine. You also need folic acid to produce S-adenosyl methionine (SAMe), an important nutrient for brain health. SAMes do several good things: they help manage your mood, help make myelin (our nerve cell insulator), and help produce melatonin, which is linked to your body's regulation of sleep.

A deficiency in B vitamins can result in fatigue; pins and needles sensations in the hands and feet; skin issues, including eczema; irritability; and flat affect (an absence or much-reduced emotional response). It is quite easy to become depleted in B vitamins due to lifestyle factors. Alcohol, refined sugars, nicotine, caffeine, and the oral contraceptive pill all deplete our bodies of the B-complex of vitamins.

But you can build up your B vitamin levels through your diet. Food sources of B vitamins include animal protein (red meat, poultry, and eggs), whole grains, dark-green leafy vegetables, nuts, and some fruits (such as bananas, watermelon, and grapefruit). However, bananas and watermelon are not recommended because they are high in sugar and can promote glycation. To augment the B vitamins you consume in your diet, you can supplement with a high-quality B-complex vitamin that includes vitamin B_{12} in a methylcobalamin form and folic acid as 5-methyltetrahydrofolate (5-MTFH).

VITAMIN D

Vitamin D is an important antioxidant and anti-inflammatory. It plays a vital role in bone health and has also been linked to lowering cancer risk, including colon and breast cancers. It can improve insulin sensitivity, further decreasing the risk of diabetes (and glycation risk). It may also strengthen our immune systems and help improve our mood during the winter months.

During this pandemic, doctors have received conflicting evidence about vitamin D's role in the body's immune response to COVID-19. Many medical teams found an association between groups at risk of vitamin D deficiency and groups at high risk of severe COVID-19, along with a complex relationship of lower socioeconomic status and nutritional status.

Yet another research team, one at Alberta Health Services, completed a literature review and concluded that there was no high-quality evidence suggesting that taking vitamin D supplements is specifically effective in preventing or treating COVID-19.[96]

Vitamin D is called our sunshine vitamin because we use the sun to manufacture it in our skin cells. Therefore, weather plays a role in our ability to produce sufficient vitamin D. Living in northern climates (such as Canada and the northern United States) and dealing with the elements of winter can impact our vitamin D level.

Getting the right dose of vitamin D depends on genetics, age, gender, race, and the environment – and can range from 2000 iu (international units) per day to upwards of 10,000 iu per day. It's essential to ingest vitamin D supplements with food; vitamin D is a fat-soluble vitamin and absorbs better with a meal.

VITAMIN C

Vitamin C is an antioxidant and a free-radical scavenger with anti-inflammatory properties. It can stimulate the growth of white blood cells, which boost cellular immunity and vascular integrity. This vitamin also serves as a cofactor in the generation of endogenous catecholamines, which include noradrenalin and adrenaline, your flight-or-fight hormones. They are secreted to support us during times of physical or emotional stress.[97] [98]

Vitamin C is a water-soluble vitamin that is thought to have beneficial effects for patients with severe and critical illnesses. Therefore, early in this pandemic, high-dose intravenous vitamin C was used in the treatment of COVID-19 (humans require more vitamin C in states of oxidative stress, including serious infections and sepsis). Unfortunately, the potential role of high doses of vitamin C in reducing inflammation and vascular injury in patients with COVID-19 has not yet been confirmed.[99]

At the time of publication, the National Institutes of Health does not recommend either for or against the use of vitamin C in the treatment of COVID-19, citing insufficient data to date.[100]

There is much that this vitamin can do in terms of improving our overall health and reducing our risk of contracting and dying from COVID. Vitamin C can prevent LDL ("bad") cholesterol from becoming stiff. As a result, it reduces your risk of cardiovascular disease. Vitamin C is an essential vitamin when it comes to collagen and elastin formation. Collagen is one of the building blocks for your connective tissue, including skin, blood vessels, bones, tendons, and joints. It's also an important vitamin for healing cuts and wounds, and it helps repair tissue and prevents aging.

The therapeutic dosing of vitamin C is unique to each individual, and you will know when you have reached your maximum dosage when you begin to experience loose stools. This is called dosing until bowel tolerance. It is prudent to note that oxalate is a by-product of vitamin C. When vitamin C is taken in higher doses, it could increase the risk of getting kidney stones (because it can trigger the transformation of calcium into a solid form from a liquid form). It may be wise for those of you who may have a predisposition to kidney stones to avoid high doses of vitamin C.

ALPHA LIPOIC ACID

We do everything we can to prevent premature aging. This includes taking antioxidants to prevent the growth of oxidants. We eat deep-colored fruits and vegetables and/or supplement with vitamins A, C, E, selenium, glutathione, and coenzyme Q10. Yes, they're all vital antioxidants.

So why is alpha lipoic acid not just another antioxidant? Alpha lipoic acid is considered the "universal antioxidant." Unlike other antioxidants, which are either water-soluble and work outside of the cell or are fat-soluble and work inside the cell, alpha lipoic acid is both water- and fat-soluble and therefore works both inside and outside of the cell. Alpha lipoic acid is a powerful antioxidant on its own, but it also has the capacity to bolster other antioxidants by enabling them to be more effectively used by the body. All of these properties play a role in slowing down the aging process and promoting better overall health.

Alpha lipoic acid is also vital to balancing your sugar levels, and it also helps lower your cholesterol, helps prevent cataracts and glaucoma, and helps improve your heart health.

Alpha lipoic acid is found in some foods, including red meat, green vegetables, and bran. For each 3-ounce (90 g) serving, beef kidney has 32 mcg of alpha lipoic acid, beef heart has 19 mcg, and beef liver has 14 mcg. One cup (250 mL) of raw spinach has 5 mcg, and the same amount of rice bran has 11 mcg. So supplementation with alpha lipoic acid would be a more convenient way to take in the recommended daily dose (300 to 600 mg) – unless, of course, you're prepared to eat 3 pounds (1.5 kg) of beef kidneys every day. Alpha lipoic acid commonly comes in 25-mg and 50-mg doses.

MAGNESIUM

Magnesium is an important trace mineral that's essential to more than 300 biochemical reactions in your body. Some of these reactions include energy production, bone-building, the synthesis of fats and antioxidants, wound healing, and the secretion of certain hormones. A magnesium deficiency can lead to several health problems, such as muscle cramping/twitching, headaches, irritability, constipation, and decreased bone strength.

But magnesium has other benefits as well. It can be used to decrease blood pressure or as a sleep aid. And it can also reduce the number of asthma attacks, and cut the risk of metabolic syndrome associated with an increased risk of diabetes.

You can develop a magnesium deficiency when you don't consume enough via your diet. But it can also occur if you exercise strenuously. When we exercise, we sweat (a vital process in keeping our bodies cool – our internal air conditioner). The downside to our "air-conditioning unit" is that it depletes our magnesium supply and triggers the symptoms I've just described.

It's important to replenish with an electrolyte replacement or magnesium tablets during exercise and after exercise. Another way we deplete our bodies of magnesium is by enjoying that fine glass of wine (or any alcohol, for that matter). Although you may not want to read this, it's true: alcohol leeches magnesium from our bodies in a dose-dependent way – meaning that the more alcohol consumed, the more depletion of magnesium.

It's important to choose the right magnesium supplement. Magnesium oxide is not recommended because it's poorly absorbed. Magnesium carbonate and magnesium citrate can help promote healthy bowels by improving constipation. But when it's used in higher doses, these can cause loose stools and should not be used if you have a tendency to experience diarrhea. Magnesium glycinate, or magnesium amino acid chelate, is usually more expensive than other forms of magnesium, but it is absorbed more easily and has fewer side effects on your bowels. Magnesium dosing varies greatly depending on the condition being targeted, so you'll want to consult with a healthcare professional to determine the right dose for you.

IRON

We need iron to transport and store oxygen. But iron plays a vital role in how our bodies produce energy too. Therefore, low levels of iron can cause fatigue, lethargy, and dizziness. An iron deficiency can also be a culprit in cold hands and feet, brain fog, and reduced immunity. An athlete with low iron levels will experience poor exercise tolerance and decreased fitness because iron is a critical nutrient contributing to hemoglobin – our red blood cells, and red blood cells are needed to carry oxygen throughout our body. Lower iron can also impede our thyroid function, lowering our metabolism. Iron is truly all about energy production.

Iron deficiency is also a risk for women in their childbearing years, pregnant women, and vegetarians and vegans. Men and postmenopausal women tend not to have iron deficiencies and should avoid iron supplementation unless their iron values have been tested. Having too much iron in your body can cause iron overload, or, as I like to refer to it, rust the body from the inside out.

Supplementing with iron can be difficult because of its side effects, which include constipation and nausea. Many of us shy away from taking iron supplements for this reason.

The strongest forms of iron are ferrous sulfate, fumarate, and glu-conate, and they're available by prescription to correct iron-deficiency anemia. However, these are usually the forms that cause negative side effects. But you can get gentler forms of iron without prescription that are non-constipating, and these include heme and nonheme forms.

Heme iron is absorbed more easily than nonheme iron but may not be an appropriate choice if you're a vegetarian because it comes from an animal source. Be smart when supplementing with iron: too much of a good thing may not, in fact, be good at all.

ZINC

Zinc is deemed an essential mineral because your body can't produce it on its own; therefore, you need to consume zinc through your diet. It is the second-most-abundant trace mineral in your body, after iron, and it's present in every cell.

Zinc is necessary for more than 300 enzymatic reactions, which aid in metabolism, growth, DNA synthesis, protein production, immune health, digestion, nerve function, and many other processes.

Zinc is also needed for your senses of taste and smell. Because one of the enzymes crucial for proper taste and smell is dependent on this nutrient, a zinc deficiency can reduce your ability to taste and smell.

Although we know that many COVID-19 patients experience a loss of taste and smell, there is no evidence suggesting that zinc supplementa-tion will prevent or help treat this viral infection; rather, zinc is helpful only in the recovery process by supporting the function of your immune cells. Scientists believe that COVID-19 causes a change in our nasopha-ryngeal zinc balance, which leads to a change in sensory function.[101]

AMINO ACIDS

There are three amino acids: arginine, glutamine, and glycine.

Arginine

Arginine is a semi-essential amino acid. Usually, your body can syn-thesize enough arginine to meet its physiological demands – although, under periods of stress, the synthesis slows. This is worrisome because arginine is responsible for facilitating wound healing and promoting the secretion of key hormones, such as insulin and glucagons. Arginine is also the precursor for synthesizing nitric oxide, which is responsible for decreasing inflammation and oxidation and boosting your blood flow capacity. Arginine also has the ability to prevent blood clotting and "stickiness."

We also know that higher doses of arginine can boost growth hormone levels, leading to stronger bones, muscle building, and tissue repair. It's also been proven that exercise and good sleep hygiene help increase growth hormone levels.

Some examples of arginine-rich foods are red meat, fish, poultry, grains, nuts, seeds, and dairy products. If you suffer from cold sores, take note: if you consume a diet rich in arginine foods, you increase your risk of cold sores. *Herpes simplex virus 1* (HSV-1) uses arginine to replicate itself. It is not recommended to use arginine supplementation if you have an increased risk for cold sores.

Glutamine

Glutamine is the amino acid responsible for providing energy to the cells that line your digestive tract. Its main job is to repair the digestive tract, especially after periods of physical stress. It has the ability to aid in muscle recovery along with arginine and can be prescribed to decrease alcohol cravings. Glutamine, along with glycine, is required to build the most powerful antioxidant of all: glutathione.

The glutamine amino acid can support the synthesis of proteins, which are the building blocks of health. This, in turn, leads to muscle building and storing glycogen as energy in the muscle. Glutamine also stabilizes our blood sugar levels by moderating insulin levels and can improve our brain function by providing glucose to brain cells. This gives our brain cells the energy they need to promote alertness, focus, and memory.

Glutamine is present in many foods, such as beans, red meat, fish, poultry, and dairy products, but it's hard to achieve therapeutic dosing from food alone. The recommended starting dose is 5 g, and to achieve that, you'll need to look at supplementation.

Glycine
The smallest and "simplest" of all the amino acids, glycine is needed to metabolize glucose, to release growth hormone, and for normal cell growth, cognitive support, and improved mood. Glycine is also useful for detoxifying many toxic influences, such as exposure to jet fuel, carpeting, dry-cleaning solvents, and gasoline.

Taking a dose of glycine can help decrease acute anxiety symptoms and decrease symptoms associated with hypoglycemia.

As with most amino acids, food sources of glycine are beans, red meat, fish, poultry, and dairy products. Glycine supplementation is a sweet-tasting powder that is most commonly dosed under the tongue for full absorption. A starting dose of glycine would be 4 g.

ACTIVE HEXOSE CORRELATED COMPOUND (AHCC)

AHCC is a highly researched proprietary mushroom extract that has been used in Eastern medicine for many centuries. It uses extracts of the mycelium (the vegetative part) of shiitake mushrooms. The glucans (active sugars) in the mushrooms have powerful immune-boosting capabilities and help the body fight viruses.[102]

AHCC focuses primarily on improving the innate immune system, or the part of your immune system that you are born with. Studies show that it can actually increase the number of readily available cell types in your immune system: natural killer cells, dendritic cells, and cytokines. These are of utmost importance for the immune system's ability to respond to infections and tumor growth.[103]

More than 30 clinical studies have researched this naturally extracted compound, with 20 human trials on the compound's effectiveness and impeccable safety profile. AHCC is commonly available as a 500-mg capsule. Dosage varies, but for general maintenance, one per day is sufficient. When I have felt a cold coming on, my naturopathic doctors have advised me to take three capsules in the morning and another three in the evening to boost my immune system. This reduces the duration and severity of my illness, allowing me to get back to work and feel better sooner.

Summary of Tests to Perform

Metabolic profile (blood spot sample)

- Fasting blood sugar
- Hemoglobin A1C
- Cholesterol panel – triglycerides, LDL, HDL
- C-reactive protein

Hormones (blood spot or saliva* sample)

- Insulin
- Growth hormone
- *Testosterone
- *Estrogen

Nutrients

- Common (blood spot)

  - Omega fatty acids
  - B vitamins (folate and B_{12} especially)
  - Vitamin D
  - Magnesium
  - Iron (stored form as ferritin)
  - Zinc

- Specialty (requires specialized labs)

  - Vitamin C
  - Alpha lipoic acid
  - Amino acids

The above tests can be performed in the comfort of your home with self-test kits.

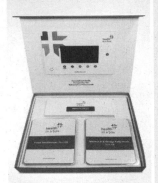

Six easy steps to a healthier you

Step 1
Order and receive your at-home test kits

Step 2
Collect and ship your samples

Step 3
Receive your results on a secure portal

Step 4
Review your results with your health professionals

Step 5
Create an action plan based on your metrics

Step 6
Get coaching support to manage change

Visit: www.healthinabox.com

CHAPTER 5

Is Your Mind in Balance?

Traditionally, the way to determine a person's state of mental health is to ask, "How are you feeling?" Since the pandemic began in March 2020, we have all been feeling a range of emotions. Many describe themselves as feeling sad, stressed, or even hyper. In fact, it's been a challenge to navigate not just our emotional states but also our physical state.

But why?

During each wave of the pandemic, our brains have sensed a threat to our survival. The enemy, the SARS-CoV-2 virus, is invisible and could be anywhere – in our workplace and even in our home. COVID-19 can be asymptomatic, but it can also kill a loved one in just days.

This anguish causes our body to go into a fight-or-flight mode, resulting in the secretion of several hormones, most notably cortisol, which triggers an adrenaline rush. As you will recall from Chapter 3, this chemical increases our heart rate and blood pressure, and it floods us with energy to get us ready to face the enemy. Yet the enemy is unclear, and so we sit nervously in our chairs, waiting for something unknown to happen.

As we learned to mask up, wash our hands, and physically distance ourselves from loved ones, colleagues, friends, and family, we developed routines that eased our fears. The acute state of anxiety and grief gave way to a chronic emotional state that is best described as languishing or floundering.

Confinement Syndrome

COVID-19 has emotionally impacted almost every single person alive. Social isolation has been one of the harshest outcomes for many people. While not as severe as prisoners who experience confinement syndrome while in solitary confinement, the restrictions and sensory deprivation many of us have experienced during this pandemic have created various physical and mental health issues.

A group of physicians in France described the impact on some long-term care residents who died not from acute respiratory distress syndrome due to COVID-19 but rather from "confinement disease."[104] These patients were left alone in their rooms for many days without help, due to worker understaffing. They died from the side effects caused by being confined to their room with nobody to feed or clean them. Hypovolemic shock (severe dehydration) was the cause of death – and totally preventable. Without human stimulation, these seniors also developed significant mental illnesses, such as delirium, depression, and suicidal ideations.

The risk of confinement syndrome increases when social networks and support systems are disrupted, including the support provided by essential caregivers and visitors in hospitals, community centers, and nursing homes. These disruptions are compounded by an imposed or voluntary reduction in travel and mobility within communities for fears of spreading and contracting the disease.

Some of the triggers of mental illnesses can be identified from neuroendocrine chemical markers. We know that some of these "brain chemicals" are implicated in depression, anxiety, obsessive-compulsive disorders, and schizophrenia.

Our neuroendocrine system is a complex set of neurons (nerve cells), glands, and nonsecretory tissues. They function in an integrated fashion to regulate our physiological and behavioral states through a combination of neurochemicals and hormones. This system begins in our brain, specifically in our hypothalamus and pituitary gland, which control the release of hormones in our body.

Hormones keep us in balance, or homeostasis, with our reproductive system, metabolism, energy, mood, and, well, just about everything – including our basic heart and respiratory rates and blood pressure.

I've often said that once we pass age 40, we've outlived our evolutionary function, which is to make babies and pass our DNA along to the next generation. Everything in our hormone soup changes dramatically around the age of 40. Often we focus on the drop of estrogen levels in women, and testosterone levels in men. For women, we call this menopause, and for men, andropause. Our muscles, bones, and tissues don't recover as quickly after injury and even after an exercise workout.

Our physical stamina, energy, and memory begin to wane. What's happening? Simply, our bodies begin to secrete lower amounts of certain hormones needed for reproduction and survival. If this is complicated by an unhealthy lifestyle, which can cause stress and obesity, our other hormones will begin to malfunction.

Let us explore some of the important hormones that affect our mental well-being.

Cortisol

Cortisol is a steroid hormone that controls a wide range of essential processes in our bodies, especially our metabolic and immune responses. It acts as an anti-inflammatory, influences memory formation, and controls salt and water balance, impacting blood pressure.

Cortisol, as a stress-response hormone, is responsible for getting our bodies ready for a fight. Our heart rate, blood pressure, and body temperature all rise to increase our metabolism in response to stress. Regardless of the source of the stress, whether it is COVID-19 or not, the response is the same.

The Epinephrine Response

The cortisol hormone is secreted from a small organ above the kidneys called the adrenal glands – specifically from the cortex, the outside portion. Almost every cell in your body contains receptors for cortisol. As one of our glucocorticoids, this hormone helps to control blood sugar levels by increasing epinephrine synthesis (discussed later in this chapter). This increases the secretion and distribution of glucose and stored energy, partly through inhibition of insulin secretion and promotion of insulin resistance. While the epinephrine response is rapid and short-lived, the cortisol effect lasts for hours and helps the body repair damage and reduce inflammation.

When my clients ask me about weight management, I often reference an article I wrote for *Canadian Business* titled "Skipping meals makes you dumb and fat." It's true. When you wake up in the morning, cortisol is secreted to get your blood pressure up and to get your heart rate going. But if you walk out of your house without breakfast, two things happen. Without food fuel, your body begins to secrete more cortisol as a stress response to being starved, and your blood sugar levels decrease, slowing down your brain function. Next, this cortisol surge gives you a sugar craving to find carbohydrates – fast food fuel. (You'll never find yourself feeling stressed and craving a hunk of meat, but certainly a chunk of chocolate or candies.) A high intake of carbohydrates can lead to obesity because insulin stores the excess sugars as fat.

Cortisol is also regulated to some degree by estrogen – which partly explains hot flashes, sweats, and palpitations during menopause. A rush of these adrenaline-like symptoms can be very debilitating during the workday and at night when you're trying to get a deep, long sleep. Chronically poor sleep can provoke additional hormonal imbalances (reducing your cortisol, growth hormone, and serotonin) – a vicious cycle.

We need to understand just how important sleep is and the implications of sleep deprivation. During certain stages of sleep, our bodies repair themselves – hence the "refreshed" feeling we have when we wake up. With sleep deprivation, we know that cortisol levels spike.[105]

Stress Makes You Fat

A client came to our clinic complaining of a rapid 10-pound (4.5 kg) weight gain over 2 to 3 months. He had always been a keen advocate of a healthy lifestyle. He exercised at least three times a week; did weights twice a week; and ate a high-protein, complex-carbohydrate, and low-fat diet. His blood work showed his morning cortisol to be less than 200 (the normal range is between 350 and 500), and his insulin level was high, at 196 (the normal range is between 40 and 80). His blood sugar level and thyroid function were both normal. He denied eating any differently, and we suggested he go on a low-carbohydrate diet for 2 weeks and then repeat his insulin test. It was still high but better, at 156.

What happened?

It turns out he had been working on a major real estate deal for the past few months and had trouble sleeping – many nights he slept only 2 to 3 hours. Not enough sleep induces cortisol as a stress response, and high cortisol keeps us awake. But as burnout occurs due to chronic sleep deprivation, the body's need to find quick food fuel increases, helping to keep a tired body running. Insulin surges and increases our absorption of any carbohydrate we consume. So, mystery solved. My client gained weight as a stress response.

What Happens If I Have Too Much Cortisol?

To understand what happens when we have too much cortisol over a prolonged period, we can look to those who have Cushing's syndrome, an abnormal condition caused by excess levels of corticosteroids and especially cortisol in the body. This disease can be caused by a wide range of factors, such as a tumor that produces too much cortisol hormone or taking certain kinds of drugs, such as prednisone. Symptoms include:

- Rapid weight gain, mainly in the face, chest, and abdomen – contrasted with slender arms and legs
- A flushed and round face

- High blood pressure
- Increased thirst and frequency of urination
- Loss of bone mass
- Skin bruising and stretch marks
- Muscle weakness
- Mood swings, anxiety, and depression

Long-term stress, however, can reduce our cortisol response – often known as adrenal fatigue or burnout. This leads to a slower immune response, which can complicate how we prevent and repair DNA damage, which, in turn, increases our risk of infection and disease. As well, with a slower metabolic rate, we have less energy, feel more tired, and burn less fat.

What Happens If I Have Too Little Cortisol?

Medical conditions resulting in too little cortisol may be due to a problem in the pituitary gland or the adrenal glands, known as Addison's disease. The onset of symptoms is often very gradual. Symptoms include:

- Fatigue
- Dizziness
- Weight loss
- Muscle weakness
- Mood changes

If you have a smartphone, you know what happens if you don't keep it charged. You can think of your cortisol levels this way as well. A fully charged smartphone battery is usually good for a full day of activities. However, if we do an unusually high amount of talking on the phone or online surfing, the battery runs out quickly and doesn't get us through the entire day.

Our bodies need recharging too. If we get a full night's sleep, we replenish our cortisol levels, and we are powered up for the day. If we don't sleep well or long enough, we begin the day exhausted and drag through our day, feeling completely burned out by nighttime.

Cortisol Curves

To determine the health of your cortisol levels, we can look at how the hormone fluctuates in your body over a period of time. With a simple collection of your saliva during the day, we can create cortisol curves that show if you are overstretched, coping, or burned out from stressors. This is a great way to see how "well" you are truly dealing with the pandemic. See these examples of cortisol curves.

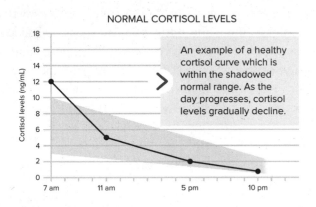

NORMAL CORTISOL LEVELS

An example of a healthy cortisol curve which is within the shadowed normal range. As the day progresses, cortisol levels gradually decline.

When you are coping "well," your cortisol levels are higher in the morning, which gets you going by stimulating your epinephrine (or adrenaline). This, in turn, increases your heart rate and blood pressure, helping all your metabolic hormones fire "go." As the day progresses, your cortisol level decreases, and so does your energy, which allows you to settle down and easily fall asleep, providing your body with the chance to rest and recover.

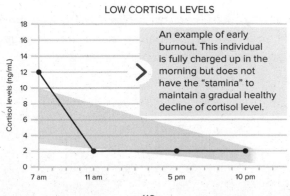

LOW CORTISOL LEVELS

An example of early burnout. This individual is fully charged up in the morning but does not have the "stamina" to maintain a gradual healthy decline of cortisol level.

This curve shows a potentially early burnout, as the cortisol is higher than ideal in the morning. The body wakes up very prepared to fight or flight. However, by the end of the morning, fatigue has set in. People often artificially improve their stamina by having a caffeinated drink (coffee, black tea, or soft drink, for example), and this beverage can mimic the effects of natural cortisol.

However, with the long-term overuse of caffeine in the morning (more than the equivalent of 2 cups/16 oz of coffee, for example) and with even more caffeine in the afternoon, you can cause your body to blunt the natural secretion of cortisol in your body. The fight-or-flight response is lost because of the caffeine. The body uses caffeine as an external stimulatory source rather than triggering the body to make a natural stimulant, cortisol, in response to stress. A flat cortisol curve resembling a burnout curve can be the result.

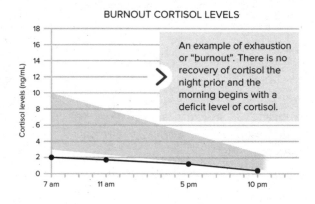

BURNOUT CORTISOL LEVELS

An example of exhaustion or "burnout". There is no recovery of cortisol the night prior and the morning begins with a deficit level of cortisol.

Certainly, those who are truly burned out from over-exhaustion and chronic stressors will also show a flat cortisol curve. The body is simply unable to produce cortisol to cope with the situation at hand.

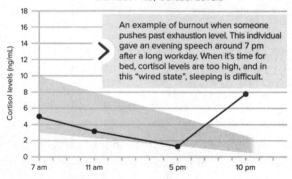

BURNING THE MIDNIGHT OIL:
Burnout Plus, Cortisol Levels

An example of burnout when someone pushes past exhaustion level. This individual gave an evening speech around 7 pm after a long workday. When it's time for bed, cortisol levels are too high, and in this "wired state", sleeping is difficult.

Too many of us keep pushing ourselves despite being exhausted. Remarkably, if the body is pushed to stay awake, the body will make more cortisol. This is likely the scenario of many essential healthcare workers who have been working night shifts during this pandemic. Unfortunately, high levels of cortisol can impair not only physical well-being but also emotional stability. Needless to say, with high cortisol, we are charged up, and it's tough to fall asleep. With insufficient quantity and quality of sleep, more negative health impacts can occur. We discuss this further in Chapter 9.

Unfortunately, there is no hormone replacement therapy for modulating cortisol response. When we are stressed or burned out, we need to moderate and change how we live. Your most important behaviors to maintain healthy cortisol levels are exercising regularly, getting good-quality sleep, and avoiding stimulants. This means that we must stay away from substances such as alcohol, caffeine, and sugar; they create a yo-yo effect of higher highs, which leads to lower lows. Other effective methods for maintaining healthy cortisol levels are daily meditation and yoga and getting a weekly massage.

In addition, with the guidance of a health practitioner, some supplements can help stabilize abnormal cortisol levels and, in essence, support your adrenal gland function. They include glandular therapies, hormone modulators, and B vitamins.

Norepinephrine (Also Known as Noradrenaline) and Epinephrine (Also Known as Adrenaline)

Both norepinephrine and epinephrine hormones are increased when the brain perceives a stressful event; therefore, they are closely connected to the expression of cortisol effects.

Naturally occurring norepinephrine is made mostly inside nerve axons (the shaft of the nerve), stored inside vesicles (small fluid-filled sacs), then released when an electrical impulse travels down the nerve. Some norepinephrine is also made from inside the medulla, the inner portion of the adrenal gland. Therefore, our adrenal medulla helps us cope with physical and emotional stress by synthesizing epinephrine from norepinephrine.

Norepinephrine increases alertness and arousal, and it speeds reaction time. Epinephrine increases during times of stress and acts on almost all body tissues. It relaxes the bronchi in our lungs, allowing for easier breathing; contracts the muscle walls of our blood vessels to increase blood pressure to our brain and heart; increases our heart rate to get more oxygen pumped around the body so that we can fight or flight; and aids in the conversion of glycogen (a stored form of energy) into glucose in the liver for fuel.

Elevated levels of these hormones can contribute to mania, anxiety, agitation, irritability, and insomnia.

Low levels of these hormones have been shown to play a role in low blood pressure, depression, and attention deficit hyperactivity disorder (ADHD), which impacts a person's ability to concentrate and focus.

Some medications have been used to help raise levels of both norepinephrine and dopamine (to be discussed later in this chapter); these include Ritalin or Concerta (methylphenidate), Dexedrine (dextroamphetamine), and Adderall (amphetamine and dextroamphetamine). Strattera (atomoxetine), another drug prescribed for ADHD, only raises levels of norepinephrine, not dopamine.

People with depression may be given a prescription from a class of drugs called serotonin-norepinephrine reuptake inhibitors (SNRIs) or selective serotonin reuptake inhibitors (SSRI).

SNRIs raise levels of both norepinephrine and serotonin in the brain. Commonly prescribed SNRIs include Effexor (venlafaxine) and Cymbalta (duloxetine).

Serotonin

I call serotonin our happiness hormone because it regulates our mood and sexual desire. As well, serotonin affects our appetite, sleep, memory, and learning. When your serotonin levels are at a normal level, you should feel focused, emotionally stable, happy, and calm.

As it gets dark each day and evening arrives, our serotonin hormone level begins to rise. Another serotonin function is to balance two neurotransmitters, dopamine and adrenaline, allowing our bodies to rest. If we were bombarded with "wakening" hormones all day, we would quickly become exhausted.

People who are deficient in this hormone often suffer from symptoms of depression, obsessive-compulsive disorder, and anxiety. Serotonin is a key hormone that triggers a hypothalamic response to secrete more ACTH (adrenocorticotropic hormone) inside the brain, which, in turn, is necessary for the release of cortisol. An insufficient supply of serotonin will lead to an insufficient release of cortisol. Therefore, it's important to ensure your serotonin levels are sufficient, to counteract the negative feelings of burnout caused by stress.

The Gut-Brain Connection

Over the past 10 years, there has been an explosion of research focused on our gut biome, the community of microorganisms (bacteria, fungi, and archaea) that live in our digestive tract. Gut bacteria produce approximately 95% of the body's supply of serotonin.[106] (We discuss the gut biome in Chapter 8.)

Researchers have confirmed that there is a strong connection between our brain and our gut. They communicate with each other by sending hormone signals to each other. Therefore, there is truth to the expressions "What a gut-wrenching decision I made" and "I have butterflies in my stomach," for example. Many don't realize that serotonin receptors are found throughout our bodies, including our bowels.

The exact level of serotonin in the brain required for positive mental health remains a mystery. Once it was discovered that there is a connection between serotonin and depression, doctors could treat this illness, in part, as a hormone disorder.

We do know that what we eat can influence our levels of serotonin. In particular, tryptophan, an amino acid that is used in making serotonin, is found in protein. Turkey, in particular, is known for its high level of tryptophan, as are nuts, milk, and other dairy products. Getting enough vitamin B_6 can affect the rate of conversion of tryptophan to serotonin.

Both tryptophan and a precursor to serotonin called 5-HTP are available through health professionals as a supplement. People who experience mild symptoms of depression or seasonal affective disorder often find them helpful in reducing the sensation of being "low" or "feeling down."

SSRIs, mentioned earlier, are a common medication used to treat depression. Prozac (fluoxetine) and Celexa (citalopram) are two examples. They work by doing what their name suggests: they slow down serotonin's breakdown, which increases the overall level of this hormone in the body.

Serotonin Syndrome

Serotonin syndrome can occur when you take medications that cause high levels of serotonin in your body. One such drug is cannabis – specifically tetrahydrocannabinol (THC), the hallucinogenic component of the plant. A small amount of THC can often be relaxing to some people, but too much can lead to severe side effects.

Symptoms range from shivering, heavy sweating, confusion, restlessness, headaches, high blood pressure, twitching muscles, and diarrhea. More severe symptoms include high fever, unconsciousness, seizures, and irregular heartbeat. Serotonin syndrome can happen to anyone, but people who genetically have trouble metabolizing THC are at higher risk.[107]

Dopamine

As noted earlier, one of the functions of serotonin is to counterbalance two neurotransmitters, dopamine and epinephrine. Dopamine has two main roles. The first is to regulate physical movement. People with Parkinson's disease often have low levels of this hormone and are frequently prescribed dopamine to reduce stiffness. The other role is to regulate our emotions, functioning as another feel-good neurotransmitter. The brain releases dopamine into the bloodstream when you are expecting pleasure from something, such as a favorite food, alcohol, drugs, gambling, shopping, or sex.

If the brain has too much dopamine, it can lead to excessive nerve cell activity, which can cause a person to develop an addiction due to a constant craving for the "high" associated with dopamine. Elevated dopamine may also result in increased worry, distrust of others, and a decreased ability to interact socially. This condition is often found in patients with attention deficit and hyperactivity.

Low dopamine ranges may be associated with anxiety, depression, difficulty concentrating, decreased libido, and obesity. Low ranges may also be associated with an increase in addictive behaviors and other stimulation-seeking activities in a bid to get that much-needed "rush."

Some people who experience low dopamine levels may not regenerate tetrahydrobiopterin (BH4), an essential cofactor for dopamine synthesis. Taking folic acid (vitamin B_6), vitamin B_3, vitamin C, molybdenum, and zinc can support this regeneration. Additionally, the production of dopamine requires vitamin D, iron, and vitamin B_6.

Gamma-Aminobutyric Acid (GABA)

Gamma-aminobutyric acid is an amino acid, a building block for proteins. In our nervous system, it acts as a neurotransmitter. GABA binds to neurons (nerve cells) to reduce their activity, inhibiting nerve transmission in the brain and creating a feeling of calmness. GABA is produced in your brain from glutamate, another amino acid that is generally abundant in the human diet. In addition to glutamate, your brain requires specific cofactors, including vitamin B_6, to synthesize GABA.

GABA creates a calmness of mood, and it reduces mental and physical stress, decreases feelings of anxiousness, reduces muscle tension, improves blood pressure, and helps induce sleep.

A growing body of research has demonstrated a correlation of low GABA levels to feelings of overthinking, anxiousness, and tension, leading to difficulty sleeping. A Harvard Medical School study found that people with chronic sleep problems had 30% lower GABA levels than people with average sleep patterns.[108]

What causes low GABA levels is not well understood. It may be a combination of factors, such as genetics, prolonged stress, not enough exercise, lack of certain nutrients, and poor gut health.

It has been shown that fermented foods rich in probiotics, such as sauerkraut, kimchi, miso, tempeh, yogurt, and kefir, can help to increase GABA levels.

Other foods that contain GABA include:

- Fish and shellfish
- Beans and lentils
- Sprouted whole grains
- Potatoes
- Tomatoes
- Seaweed
- Berries

Certain herbs are considered GABA activators and can help support your brain's natural production of GABA by gently activating GABA receptors. They include kava, ashwagandha, valerian, and passionflower.

Because GABA is an amino acid, it is available as a dietary supplement. It's been shown to effectively ease anxiousness and promote deep, restful sleep without side effects at 300 mg taken before bed.[109]

An increasing number of studies are currently underway to research the use of cannabis and its major nonintoxicating component cannabidiol (CBD) as a treatment for mental health and neurodevelopmental disorders. It appears that CBD modulates the effect of GABA receptors in our bodies.

In a study using MRI to observe GABA activity, CBD increased GABA levels across all brain regions.[110]

At the beginning of this chapter, I mentioned the word *languishing*. A *New York Times* article described this emotion best.

Definition of Languishing

lang-gwi-shing

It's a sense of being joyless and aimless. A condition where we feel a sense of stagnation and emptiness, a sort of middle ground of the mental health continuum, where depression is at one end of the spectrum and flourishing is at the other.[111]

Clearly, increased stress due to this pandemic has pushed many more people to feel joyless and aimless and perhaps suffer from clinical anxiety and depression. This chapter reinforces the importance of our brain's chemical function and how we need to monitor it with testing and support its proper balance with healthy eating, proper exercise, and better sleep.

Summary of Tests to Perform

Hormone:

- Cortisol – fasting (saliva test)
- Cortisol curve (saliva test)

Neurotransmitters (urine test):

- Epinephrine/adrenaline
- Norepinephrine/noradrenaline
- Serotonin
- Dopamine
- GABA

The above tests can be performed in the comfort of your home with self-test kits. Visit: www.healthinabox.com.

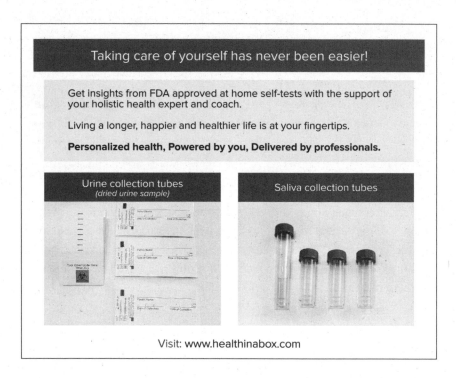

In the next section of this book, let's focus on repairing your physical and mental well-being. Once you have measured your vital signs and your physical and psychological health biomarkers, you can begin to focus on areas of concern. How can you improve your numbers? Are there science-based ways to downregulate undesired biochemical effects by detoxifying your body? Are there proactive approaches to make you less prone to the effects of stress?

REPAIRING THE DAMAGE

CHAPTER 6

How to Detox Your Body

What does it really mean to detox in the 21st century? For centuries, many civilizations have tried different methods of eliminating toxins from their bodies in the hopes of living a longer and healthier life. We are still trying to find that holy grail today.

Traditional Chinese medicine (TCM) is a branch of medicine based on the theory that energy (qi) flows through the body along pathways or energy channels, called meridians. When these meridians become unbalanced or blocked, illness occurs. TCM embraces a more holistic approach to well-being compared to Western medicine, although the gap is narrowing.

When a person's natural detox channels are not functioning well, TCM practitioners use various techniques to revitalize them with external forces, such as acupuncture, cupping, moxibustion, tui na massage, tai chi exercise, and meditation. There has been a long Chinese tradition of focusing on the health of the liver, colon, kidneys, and lungs. Today, we know these organs – along with our skin – are important in removing toxins from our bodies.

TCM focuses on seven techniques for detoxifying and promoting the body's natural healing systems.

1. Purging, forcing toxins out of the body
2. Perspiring by physical or medicinal means

3. Heat-clearing techniques
4. Replenishing
5. Warming the body
6. Eliminating toxins by urine or feces
7. Harmonizing the body

> In TCM, the concept of yin and yang represents a foundation for understanding health, including illness and wellness, focusing on the idea that life is composed of two opposite but mutually connected forces. For example, yin represents the female, darkness, rest, and right, while yang represents the male, light, activity, and left. Yin and yang are in constant flux. If one changes, so, too, must the other. These changes are usually harmonious, but sometimes they can become imbalanced, and illness occurs.

"The qi is an expression of the natural order of life. The qi always precedes the form. There is no form if there is no qi."[112]

— *Elisabeth Rochat de la Vallée, author of*
A Study of Qi in Classical Texts.

Acupuncture

The practice of acupuncture was first developed in China more than 3,000 years ago and has withstood the test of time. Today, acupuncture is commonly practiced as a routine treatment in China, Japan, Korea, and Taiwan, and since the 1970s has gained popularity in many other parts of the Western world.

Acupuncture involves the insertion of fine needles into the skin. The needles break the skin's barrier and trigger the body's natural healing response, stimulating energy flow to the body.

It's one of the fastest-growing evidence-based practices among complementary medicine practitioners. It is now a widely accepted treatment within integrative healthcare. I have recommended it to my patients as a treatment to manage pain and stress, and even for antiaging as a facial beauty service.

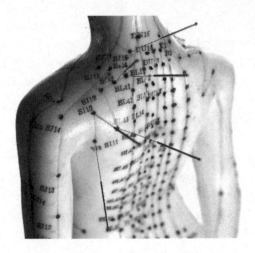

There is scientific evidence to show that acupuncture:

- Reduces pain caused by strained muscles, tendons, and nerve-pinching conditions
- Relieves tension-related headaches
- Reduces stress and anxiety to improve mood
- Supports the treatments for eating disorders and addictions such as smoking
- Improves digestion and promotes good gut health
- Reduces hot flashes and night sweats
- Increases energy

The World Health Organization lists 31 medical conditions that can be effectively treated with acupuncture.[113]

Perhaps the question many people ask is: How does acupuncture work?

As a physician educated in anatomy, physiology, and biochemistry, it is a tricky question to answer, to simply explain how a tiny, thin needle inserted at a site remote from its desired application can do so much. As an example, curing a headache by applying some needles into the leg.

There are ongoing studies that point to acupuncture's impact on our nervous system and its feedback to the brain, where signals cause the release of many hormones, impacting all our organ systems, as we've discussed in Chapters 4 and 5.

Acupuncture points are located at sites around the body and have a high density of neurovascular structures found between or at the edges of muscle groups. These locations have been identified through thousands of years of trial and error, and they are less painful than random needle sticks into a muscle group.[114]

In one study, researchers used a radioactive tracer, Technetium-99m, to see how acupuncture works in the body. The isotope was injected into both true and sham acupoints, and its movement was monitored in the body. Researchers found a random diffusion of the tracer around the sham acupoint but a rapid aggregation of the tracer along the body's meridian lines that were inconsistent with either lymphatic/vascular flow or nerve conduction pathways.[115] This study confirms the notion that acupoints do follow the energy lines within our bodies.

Modern Detoxification Modalities

Since the COVID-19 pandemic hit, we have begun to spend more time exploring ways to quickly become more resilient to emerging pathogens and for ways to recover promptly if we do get sick. Unfortunately, quick fixes are not realistic. If a person has a preexisting health condition or is obese, that person can't quickly reverse their health status in a matter of weeks or months to reduce their higher risk to COVID-19. Poor states of health rarely develop overnight.

New processed foods are added to our grocery store shelves every day, tempting shoppers to choose these over the whole, healthier options for the sake of convenience but at the expense of nutrition. News stories outlining all the types of toxins in our food are published regularly, from tainted beef to antibiotics in our meat, mercury in our fish to chemicals on our fruits and vegetables. Therefore, there has been substantial growth in the organics market, but these options are more expensive and not available to everyone.

Beyond foods, we also worry about lead in our children's toys, smog in the air, pollutants in rivers and lakes, radioactivity emitting from devices, and synthetic chemicals with unknown properties all around us.

Detoxing is an essential practice for our health. But do the more modern detox practices really offer the benefits as claimed?

In today's medical world, we use the word *detoxification* in the context of removing dangerous, often life-threatening, levels of alcohol, drugs, or poisons from our body. There are a few different kinds of treatments.

- Charcoal is often used in the emergency department to treat people who have overdosed from alcohol, drugs, and medications. The patient drinks liquid charcoal to help absorb these substances in the stomach, and then a stomach lavage is performed to pump out the drugs.
- Chelation is a type of treatment that uses intravenous or oral medications to bind to toxins, such as heavy metals, to neutralize their chemical effect. The body then eliminates them through the liver and kidney.
- Hyperbaric chambers are used to treat people with carbon monoxide poisoning by increasing pure oxygen air pressure to two to three times higher than normal, which speeds the replacement of carbon monoxide with oxygen in the body.
- A simple blood donation is a modern way of bloodletting to remove high iron levels by getting the body to lose blood and use its iron stores to make new hemoglobin.

However, in our social-media-crazed world, the word *detox* often refers to doing something quickly to try to rid ourselves of the toxins that are causing everything from weight gain, headaches, bloating, joint pain, fatigue, and depression. The "too good to be true" edict applies to many quick-fix detox methods.

Before reviewing some of the more popular detox procedures and products, let's talk about our body's natural detoxification systems.

Genetics of Detoxification

Our bodies metabolize and eliminate toxins by transforming them into a water-soluble state so that they can be excreted as feces from our colon, urine from our kidneys, and sweat from our skin. Genetics account for much of our quantitative and qualitative ability to detoxify.

Therefore, you should have genetics testing done to determine if you have any malfunctioning detoxification genes. Knowing this information allows an expert health professional to target the weakened pathway and provide a workaround. Key nutrients should also be measured, as a normal gene may also malfunction when there is a nutrient deficiency.

Genetics determines our body's ability to perform the two phases of detoxification. Phase 1 breaks apart big toxins into polar molecules. This breaking apart is called metabolism, and the substance that is formed is called a metabolite.

Phase 2 detoxification involves taking the metabolites from Phase 1 and transforming them into an excretable form. Some Phase 1 metabolites are carcinogenic or reactive, so it's very important that the Phase 2 detoxification process is functioning properly and is in sync with the first phase.

Critical to these phases are important nutrients, which function as cofactors. They include antioxidants, amino acids, and minerals – all found in a balanced and diverse diet that includes lots of vegetables and fruits.

Endogenous Detoxification Systems

Our bodies are naturally bombarded by external toxins and internal ones. External toxins are man-made, and internal toxins result from your body's natural process of metabolism, driven by our genetics. The factories in our society add to the pollutant loads in our air, earth, and water, just as our bodies' mitochondria (the "factories" in our bodies) produce toxins. We produce energy and fuel from the foods we eat. Without these internal endogenous processes, we would not survive; for example, our muscles require power to help our heartbeat, and our diaphragm expands our lungs to bring oxygen into the body and push carbon dioxide out.

We tend to forget that the body possesses many well-developed detoxification systems of checks and balances that help keep us healthy

– our body can prevent the sun's radiation from mutating our DNA, and can convert excess oxygen molecules (which could transform into dangerous superoxide or hydrogen peroxide) into harmless water. Our body does a great job so long as we nourish it with essential nutrients.

Our Detoxifying Organs

Skin. Our largest organ provides a barrier against so many harmful substances, from bacteria and viruses to heavy metals, chemical toxins, and even radiation from the sun.

Lungs. Our entire respiratory system begins with our nose, which contains tiny hairs that trap dirt and other inhaled particles. These are expelled from the airways with the help of mucus in our lung linings.

Intestines. It is not yet fully understood how this complex system works symbiotically with our gut biome. Our stomach acids kill many bacteria. The lymph nodes in the small intestine manage foreign substances before nutrients reach the colon, where they are absorbed into the blood.

Liver. This organ produces many enzymes that regulate drug metabolism, and it plays an integral part in defending our body against harmful chemicals and other toxins. It also makes a family of proteins called metallothioneins (also found in the kidneys), which metabolize dietary nutrients like copper and zinc and neutralize harmful metals like lead, cadmium, and mercury so they can be eliminated.

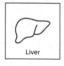

Kidneys. This organ is one of the essential filters in the body. It maintains a vigorous balance of water and minerals, such as sodium, calcium, phosphorus, and potassium, in your blood. Although these minerals can be deadly to our bodies in high quantities, we need them for a healthy metabolism.

Immune system. This network of cells (including white blood cells), antibodies, and molecules eliminates bacteria, viruses, and parasites from the body.

Immune System

Despite having intrinsic organs that already function to detoxify our bodies, we still try to live healthier and ultimately longer. Let's explore some more popular detoxification ideas.

Detox Diet or Cleanse

As a physician trained in the allopathic world, the concept of diet cleanses seemed at first strange. But over the 30-plus years of my career, I've warmed up to them – so long as they do not cause extreme harm to our bodies. The reality is that people don't eat well, and our diets are not balanced with healthy nutrition. Our brain craves many foods that are not good for our organs, beginning with sugar, caffeine, and alcohol.

The traditional idea behind cleanses is eliminating toxins by eliminating solid foods or specific food groups from our diet. This gives our digestive system a break from many unhealthy foods, allowing it to heal, repair, and absorb our nutrients more efficiently. In principle, it sounds like a great idea so long as we are not starving our bodies of other foods that are important to metabolism for an extended period of time.

Solid foods are often replaced with drinks like water with lemon, maple syrup, and cayenne pepper; green tea; or freshly squeezed fruit and vegetable juices with no solids. Cleanses can last from a day to a month. These cleanses are usually low in calories and low in protein, which will, unfortunately, leave you with little energy to exercise, an activity that is important to good health. Because there is not much fiber in these protocols, you may experience gastrointestinal discomfort. What's worse, a lack of fiber starves your gut biome. This type of "diet" is not sustainable, and depending on your level of activity, it may cause nutrient deficiencies and disrupt your metabolic rate and blood glucose levels.

Many studies have shown that fasts and extremely low-calorie diets lower the body's basal metabolic rate to conserve energy. During this time, weight is lost but not the right type of weight. Generally, lean body mass (muscle and bone) is reduced rather than fat. People who follow very low-calorie diets (800 or fewer) develop gallstones due to a sudden change in fat metabolism.

Once a more "normal" diet returns, rapid weight gain follows. Unfortunately, much of the weight lost through caloric-restricted diets results from fluid loss related to deficient carbohydrate intake and frequent bowel movements or diarrhea caused by saltwater and laxative tea.[116]

Supplements

It's best to enlist the supervision of a health professional who knows how to support clients through cleanses, as they can also add supplements to the regimen. The most common supplements associated with detoxification include vitamin C, acidophilus, psyllium husk, and herbs such as milk thistle, dandelion, turmeric, Jerusalem artichoke, and licorice root. According to my naturopathic doctor colleagues, here's why we need to take them while detoxifying.

- Vitamin C: This water-soluble antioxidant is necessary for any detoxification protocol.
- Acidophilus and other probiotics: These help to repopulate the intestinal tract with healthy ("good") gut bacteria that are crucial to proper digestion and aid in the excretion of toxic substances.
- Psyllium husk: A fiber that removes accumulated waste effectively.
- Bitter herbs (milk thistle, dandelion, turmeric, Jerusalem artichoke): Toxins released from the liver are secreted into the bile for excretion through the bowels. These bitter herbs are excellent for promoting bile flow, thus enhancing detoxification.
- Licorice root: This important herb is a potent antioxidant and anti-inflammatory, and it has antimicrobial effects.

We will discuss more science-backed diets that help with weight loss, support lowering cholesterol, and improve blood pressure in Chapter 8.

Intestinal Cleanse

This type of detoxification protocol ranges from high-fiber-laxative protocols to self-administered enemas to "medical" colonic procedures. The goal is to remove toxins from your gut, which is thought to be dirty with stool.

Like fasting, colonic cleanses carry a risk of dehydration, electrolyte imbalance, impaired bowel function, and disruption of intestinal flora.

In the past 10 years, our views of stool have changed in the medical world. We've discovered that the gut is important to functions other than absorbing nutrients and water. It also houses many types of "good" bacteria, which work symbiotically with our body to ensure we remain healthy from parasites and to help improve our mood (as discussed earlier with serotonin production in Chapter 5). During COVID-19, there has been far more discussion among scientists about the importance of the gut biome supporting the immune system. Therefore, "washing out" the good bacteria along with the bad simply does not make sense.

Gut Biome

There are 100 million times more bacteria on Earth than there are stars in the universe. We likely know more about our stars than our gut biome. Most of the cells in our bodies are not our own cells but are comprised of bacteria that colonize in our bodies. Particularly in the gut and colon, trillions of bacteria coexist in harmony with your other cells. The term *gut microbiome* is used to describe this bacterial collective. This is a relatively new concept in the allopathic doctor community that we are just beginning to learn about; our progress in this area mirrors how we were slow to embrace genetics into daily practice more than 10 years ago.

An average person has about 3 pounds (1.5 kilograms) of gut bacteria. Since birth, your body has evolved along with a collection of guest bacteria that build and shape you. Your microbiome is crucial in protecting you against pathogens, maintaining a healthy immune system, and helping you absorb your nutrients from food.

We now know that your gut biome plays a role in conditions like ulcerative colitis, Crohn's disease, irritable bowel syndrome (IBS), and even heart disease and depression. These bacteria impact how hungry you are and how much you weigh.

What we eat can change the balance of microbes in our digestive tracts. Choosing between a bacon, lettuce, and tomato (BLT) sandwich versus just a salad with lean protein for lunch will increase the populations of some types of bacteria and diminish others. As their numbers change, they secrete different substances, activate different genes, and absorb various nutrients. Therefore, your food choices influence your gut biome, which, in turn, impacts your health.

Our gut biome feeds on prebiotics, which are nondigestible plant-based fibers – from foods like apples, onions, garlic, bananas, and oats – that pass through the gastrointestinal tract. However, when we eat a high-sugar diet, the undesirable bacteria thrive and start to grow out of control, while our beneficial bacteria dwindle in number.

An emerging body of research suggests that our food cravings may be significantly shaped by the bacteria we have inside our gut. They influence our reward and satiety pathways, produce toxins that alter mood, make changes to receptors (including taste receptors), and alter our vagus nervous system, the neural axis between the gut and the brain.[117]

Unfortunately, our modern lifestyles challenge our gut biome every day, not only with our diets full of sugar and processed chemicals but also from antibacterial items, like prescription antibiotics (which damage our gut's flora population), medications, and alcohol absorbed from alcohol-based hand sanitizers (which we are now using in the gallons during this pandemic). Contaminants in our water and food and even stress induced by the pandemic can change the balance of good versus bad gut flora.

Acid blockers, which are taken for reflux, also impact gut bacteria. They stop the acidity in your stomach, lower the pH level, and kill your "good" gut flora. Therefore, it's essential to recognize that *everything we ingest* impacts our physical and mental health.

Because our gut biome is so crucial to our physical health and our mental well-being, I'm not an advocate for intestinal cleanses since they wash out our good and bad gut bacteria, which are difficult to rebuild back with prebiotics and probiotics.

Gut Permeability

For many years, I took medications to treat reflux. When I was finally able to test my microbiome population, I discovered very low biodiversity of biome species in my gut. As naturopathic doctors would say, this increased my overall gut permeability, which causes an increased incidence of gastrointestinal symptoms, ranging from gas and bloating to cramps and diarrhea. Far too often, I can get food poisoning–like symptoms from a meal that I've shared with others who do not experience the same symptoms. This experience supports my case that my gut is "weak." Today I continue to work hard to keep my gut happier, with lots of prebiotic foods and probiotics. It continues to be a never-ending battle.

Enemas and colonics are popular in some circles. I can unequivocally say: *Do not do it.* There is no merit in pumping fluids into the lower bowel to cause irritation of the gut and create a lower bowel purging of your stool. Along with actual toxins and by-products of digestion, you also eliminate your entire gut flora. The only time we have no choice but to do an oral purge is to prepare for a colonoscopy to look for bowel cancer. It is acceptable to endure this procedure once every few years, since it can save your life.

Fecal Transplants

Medical doctors are now researching fecal microbiota transplants (FMT), which show some effectiveness in treating some colon diseases. Fecal transplantation is a medical procedure that involves inserting stool from a healthy donor into a recipient to restore the normal microbiome inside their large bowel. An FMT is performed in a medical environment by a medical specialist. Healthy donors are first screened for bacterial, viral, or parasitic infections to ensure that dangerous microorganisms are not introduced to the patient receiving the FMT. There have been positive results in treating patients with recurrent infections from a common, hospital-acquired bacteria known as *Clostridium difficile*.[118]

A groundbreaking 2015 study done at McMaster University in Hamilton, Canada, showed dramatic results with FMT. It was the first to show that fecal transplants can improve symptoms of ulcerative colitis.[388] The Pediatric Fecal Microbiota Transplant for Ulcerative Colitis (PediFETCh) study will help determine whether fecal transplants can be a viable treatment for children who have this condition but can't control their disease with their current medication.

Oxygen Detox

Perhaps you've seen oxygen bars in Las Vegas or watched professional athletes inhale oxygen on the sidelines during their football or basketball games. The goal is to deliver air containing a high oxygen concentration (85% to 95%) through a mask or nasal tube. Concentrated oxygen has been used to boost the immune system, relieve headaches, increase energy, and improve cognitive function. Normal air in the atmosphere has a mixture of oxygen and other gases. Inhaled air by volume contains about 78% nitrogen, 21% oxygen, and small amounts of other gases, including argon, carbon dioxide, neon, helium, and hydrogen.[119]

Historically, pressurized oxygen has been widely used in medical settings to treat people experiencing respiratory distress or who have chronic lung conditions, such as emphysema and chronic obstructive pulmonary disease (COPD). Their diseased lungs cannot extract enough oxygen from room air. And pressurized oxygen has been in the news during the pandemic as well. Intensive care units are using ventilators daily in the fight against pneumonia caused by COVID-19. Ventilators push concentrated oxygen into the lungs to help patients get higher levels of oxygen into their bloodstream.

There is no evidence that healthy lungs need a higher oxygen concentration than is in normal air to supply the body with adequate oxygen. Although there is little danger from inhaling unpressurized concentrated oxygen (versus pressurized from ventilators), the FDA has cautioned against the use of "flavored" oxygen, which may contain fragrant oil suspensions that can irritate or even damage the lungs. This warning is in line with concerns about flavored vaping pods.

> It is illegal to administer oxygen from a tank without a prescription. Still, most jurisdictions have failed to enforce this FDA ruling, enabling oxygen bars to thrive.

Halotherapy and Salt Therapy

Halo is the Greek word for "salt." Halotherapy treatment involves breathing salty air either in a dry or wet format.

The dry method is often delivered in a man-made, humidity-free salt cave. A halogenerator grinds salt into microscopic particles and releases them into a cool room set to 68°F (20°C) or lower. Some people own Himalayan salt lamps, but they do not generate any salt particles. They do, however, look beautiful in a room.

The principle of this dry therapy is to experience negative ions produced by salt.

Supporters claim these salt particles absorb irritants, including allergens and toxins, from the respiratory system, reducing mucus and inflammation and resulting in clearer airways. These salt particles are said to have a similar effect on your skin.

There is no solid science to back these claims. I would categorize dry halotherapy as a relaxing spa treatment with a positive placebo effect to improve our mood, given it's often a room where many spa-goers sit after they have had a relaxing body treatment.

However, we do have evidence that the topical use of a mixture comprised of salt and water is helpful in some situations. Doctors recommend this mixture to treat many types of infection, including pink eye, skin cuts, and infected gums. Nasal lavage for sinus infections has also been helpful for many who suffer from painful congested sinuses.

During the summer of 2020, some researchers proved that introducing saltwater-based rinses into the nasal cavity decreased the viral burden through the physical removal of the SARS-CoV-2 virus.[120]

Lymphatic Drainage Massage

The lymphatic system is part of our immune system and is comprised of tissues, vessels, and organs (lymph nodes, spleen, thymus, and tonsils). About 5.3 gallons (20 L) of plasma flow through the main arterial portion of our circulatory system. Then 4.5 gallons (17 L) are returned through our veins. The remaining 0.8 gallons (3 L) seep through small capillaries into our body's tissues. Our lymphatic system collects this excess fluid, which is now called lymph, and eventually returns it back into our circulatory system.

Lymph contains lymphocytes (a type of white blood cell), which fight bacteria, viruses, and fungi. This system is also critical in our fight against COVID-19. Lymph fluid also maintains body fluid levels, absorbs digestive tract fats, and removes cellular waste.

Lymphatic drainage massage or treatment is not a deep-tissue massage. In contrast, it is gentle, using repetitive strokes to move lymph along the lymphatic system. It is a specialized massage that is sometimes referred to as a detox massage.

Health conditions such as infection and cancer, plus some medical treatments, can cause lymph fluid to build up in a particular area of the body, often in the arms or legs, causing swelling, also known as lymphedema. Lymphatic massage can improve circulation and hence lymph fluid movement to reduce swelling. It might be more effective than connective tissue massage in relieving symptoms of stiffness and depression in people living with fibromyalgia, where the cause of this condition is not well understood.[121]

Hydrotherapy

Many cultures have used water as a religious experience and a form of medical therapy for many centuries. There is scientific support for the use of water as a treatment at various temperatures, which can produce different effects on different body systems. A review of published studies suggests that these effects are scientifically documented, but the mechanisms are still being researched.

We have all used cold compresses after an injury, which reduces pain due to swelling.[122] These effects are well accepted. Bathing in water also has physiological effects, and it has been shown to reduce stress and inflammation.

One hour of bathing in water at various temperatures produces various effects. Immersion at 89.6°F (32°C) did not change metabolic rate or body temperature. However, bathing does lower heart rate (by 15%), systolic blood pressure (by 11%), and diastolic blood pressure (by 12%), compared with controls in room-air temperatures. Notably, our stress hormone, cortisol, dropped by 34%, proving that a warm bath indeed does reduce stress.

Immersion at 68°F (20°C) produced similar results, lowering heart rate, blood pressure, and cortisol levels. But this temperature caused an increase in metabolic rate by 93%.

With even colder water, at 57.2°F (14°C), the body temperature lowered, and metabolic rate significantly increased by 350%. Heart rate and blood pressure dropped by only 5% and 8%, respectively. Not surprisingly, bathing in cool water can cause panic to some degree, thereby increasing plasma noradrenaline and dopamine concentrations by 530% and 250%, respectively.[123]

And even frigid water seems to have some positive effects. Regular cold-climate swimming has been shown to significantly decrease tension and fatigue, improve memory, reduce negative mood, and relieve pain.[124]

For our practical purposes, water therapy simply does work.

Hydrotherapy has been effectively used to improve many conditions, including congestive heart failure, post-recovery of myocardial infarction, chronic obstructive pulmonary diseases, asthma, Parkinson's disease, ankylosing spondylitis, rheumatoid arthritis, osteoarthritis, fibromyalgia, anorectal disorders, fatigue, anxiety, obesity, hypercholesterolemia, hyperthermia, and labor. It has also been shown to boost immunity and help manage pain.[125]

Although I can't see doctors in hospitals using this form of treatment in acute COVID-19 patients, I can see hydrotherapy used to treat post-COVID-19 patients suffering from complications related to their infection.

Sauna

At the beginning of the chapter, we identified sweating as a form of detoxification through our skin's pores. Saunas have been used for thousands of years and are still popular today, most recently using infrared lights.

The Mayan people used sweathouses 3,000 years ago. Native Americans have also used various forms of ritual cleansing and purification, such as the sauna-like sweat lodge, for many centuries.

There are several types of saunas, differentiated by how the room is heated.

Modern saunas generate dry heat from an electrical source in the room, while older forms of saunas burn wood to generate heat. Temperatures can reach 150°F to 176°F (65°C to 80°C). Infrared saunas use infrared lamps to create heat but do not heat the air. These lamps warm the body directly and operate at a lower room temperature: 122°F to 140°F (50°C to 60°C).

A steam room uses moist heat and high humidity to increase your body's temperature and to cause you to sweat.

While there are several studies on traditional dry-heat saunas, there are few studies completed that look specifically at infrared saunas, which have become more popular in the past 10 years. I believe all saunas have similar benefits. They include:

- Better sleep
- Relaxation
- Relief from sore muscles

- Relief from joint pain
- Clearer and tighter skin
- Improved circulation

When our body temperature increases, the diameter of the blood vessels increases (vasodilates), and our heart rate increases, improving circulation. This can lower blood pressure and mimics a kind of passive exercise, especially for those who have medical reasons and cannot do an aerobic workout.

A Finnish study followed 2,315 men ages 42 to 60 over 20 years. They found a correlation between sauna use and a decrease in the risk of dying from cardiovascular disease. Those who used the sauna two to three times per week were 22% less likely to experience a sudden fatal heart attack than those who used it only once a week. As well, those who used a sauna four to seven times a week were 63% less likely to experience sudden cardiac death and 50% less likely to die from cardiovascular disease than those who used a sauna only once a week.[126]

It's often said that what is good for the heart is good for the brain. With improved cardiovascular health, both organs stay healthy. Therefore, it is significant but not surprising that another Finnish research paper using the same cohort noted above outlined a promising link between sauna use and lowering the lifetime risk for dementia and late Alzheimer's disease. It found that those who used a sauna two to three times per week were 22% less likely to develop dementia and 20% less likely to develop Alzheimer's disease than those who did not use a sauna. And those who used a sauna four to seven times a week were 66% less likely to develop dementia and 65% less likely to develop Alzheimer's disease than those who used a sauna once a week.[127]

However, this longitudinal study does not prove that taking saunas reduces cardiac and dementia risks. People who take regular saunas likely have other healthy habits that contribute to their overall health.

There are other benefits of sauna bathing as well. We know that while we sit quietly in a sauna, we relax (so long as the heat is comfortable). Our stress response decreases as our cortisol hormone level lowers. Because cortisol plays a pivotal role in oxidation and inflammation, a lower level may reduce arthritis pain, improve asthma flare-ups, and improve skin conditions such as psoriasis.[128]

Supporting Detoxification with Lifestyle

Once we understand the genetics of detoxification, we can better determine what additional factors we can add to our way of life to improve the functions of our detox pathways, beginning with a good diet (see Chapter 8 for more information). Several additional steps can be taken:

Fasting: Consuming fewer toxins can help all our organs recover. While there are many fasting diets in circulation, let's start with a few simple things. Eliminate alcohol, caffeine, sugar, and reactional drugs.

Supplements: Many products can support the functions of the liver and kidney, discussed in this chapter.

Regular elimination: One of the best things to put in your body is ample amounts of water! This helps keep you regular and drives toxins out of your body. In addition to water, we need fiber to regularly move our bowels and feed our gut biome to function correctly.

Improving circulation: Blood delivers nutrients to our cells and removes toxins and metabolites. A strong heart and good blood pressure is a great beginning. This can be achieved with regular exercise.

In the next chapter, I discuss how to de-stress by healing the mind through holistic means.

CHAPTER 7

How to De-Stress

Stress Is Our Number-One Enemy

In 2007, the World Health Organization (WHO) identified stress as one of the world's top health risks, rising significantly even in developing countries. Study after study has directly linked stress to many health issues, such as cardiovascular disease, cancer, and certainly anxiety and depression.[129] [130] Today, stress is now the most prevalent global disease of our time, no thanks to the pandemic. Hardly anyone has been spared.

Even before the pandemic, stress in the workplace has been top of mind for many HR (human resource) leaders in organizations worldwide. As we discussed in Chapter 2, lockdowns, sudden changes in work styles, and managing the risks of COVID-19 in the workplace, especially essential workers, have pushed so many people over the edge.

The opposite of feeling stressed is feeling well. Holistic well-being reflects four interconnected variables: financial, physical, mental, and social health. The insurance company MetLife has been surveying employees from the many companies they insure for almost 20 years. Their April 2021 report[131] found that more than half of the employees feel worried about at least one of these variables. Not surprisingly, stressors and challenges have more adversely impacted people of color and younger generations.

Essential workers are far more worried about their well-being compared to nonessential workers, especially about their physical health.

Here are the statistics that scream out that stressors during the pandemic have caused an increase in distress, compared to a year ago, in April 2020.

We often say we are stressed when we experience unrelenting agitation or exhaustion, or we feel burned out. With more severe stress, some feel fear and helplessness. As we described earlier, lower cortisol levels – which can be caused by chronic stress – can impact many parts of our body, especially our immune system.

In a study of medical students, researchers found that their immunity decreased, especially during stressful exams. The students had fewer natural killer cells, which fight tumors and viral infections. The medical students also stopped producing immunity-boosting gamma interferon and experienced weakly functioning T cells, which fight infection.[132]

I can personally relate to the findings of this study! For many years during university, I would come down with a cold or feel sick a few days after final exams. It seemed acceptable to me at the time, but today, I know better. It is not good for my health in the long term.

Earlier in the book, we talked about the impacts of the pandemic and social isolation. This, in turn, has caused many people to experience depression. Depression has also been shown to impact our immune health. Even mild depression can lead to a chronic reduction of T-cell function. A study showed that the duration of depression, rather than the severity, more severely impacted the immune system.[133]

Mind–Body Connection

I've weaved together many scientific details in earlier chapters to demonstrate that our mind truly controls our body. We physically experience stress because our brain tells our adrenal gland to secrete cortisol, which then secretes epinephrine.

In Chapter 5, we discussed the effects of epinephrine. It speeds up our heart rate and breathing. Often, we say we feel panicked. When our stress is not acute, chronic low epinephrine levels cause our muscles to tighten and our blood pressure to rise. We feel tense because we are!

The Secret to De-Stressing Is to Lower Our Cortisol

In following chapters, we will discuss in more detail how to maintain a healthy cortisol level by having better lifestyle habits. Other effective methods for maintaining healthy cortisol levels are weekly massages, daily meditation, yoga, and engaging in less traditional forms of contemplative practices and therapy, such as tai chi and qigong.

Massage

Many of us have likely experienced a massage and other body services offered at a spa. These services are often the first go-to physical means to de-stress. It feels great while we are on the massage table and for hours afterward, yet we rarely speak about the impact on our biochemistry.

One review article looked at a number of medical studies that used massage therapy to address specific health conditions, including depression, pain syndromes, autoimmune diseases, job stress, and pregnancy. Unequivocally, the data revealed improvements in three hormones important in how we perceive stress.

Massage therapy decreased cortisol by 31% and activated two neurotransmitters: serotonin (our "happy" hormone) increased by 28% and dopamine (our "satisfaction" hormone) by 31%.[134]

It's important to make massage a regular part of your lifestyle because it is medically effective in alleviating stress.

Meditation and Mindfulness Training

Buddhists have long practiced meditation and mindfulness to, among other reasons, reduce psychological stress and promote well-being. And modern Western medicine is catching up with the practice. I would encourage you to try these types of contemplative practices to better cope with and recover from the effects of the pandemic.

In a landmark study, meditation improved the attention skills of the participants. Enhancing task-relevant attention and focus rather than straying toward uncertainties and the difficulties of day-to-day stress-ors enabled those who meditated to be better able to perceive stressful life circumstances and thoughts as less threatening, thereby reducing psychological and physiological stress.

In other words, you can train your mind to focus on certain feelings and thoughts and on staying in the present, rather than constantly having negative thoughts about the past or future. Focusing on the "now" creates a more active problem-solving perspective on your life, compared to a more passive thought pattern that includes unease and self-doubt.[135, 136]

Richard Lazarus and Susan Folkman's Stress and Coping Theory defines coping as "constantly changing (moment to moment) cognitive and behavioral efforts to manage the demands of a stressful situation."

If you evaluate a situation and believe there is a good chance you can control it, this will induce you to find a more active solution-focused

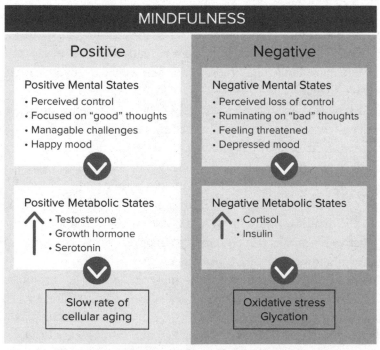

Source: Adapted from Can meditation slow rate of cellular aging? Cognitive stress, mindfulness, and telomeres, by Epel E, Daubenmier J, Moskowitz JT, Folkman S, and Blackburn E. Ann N Y Acad Sci. 2009 Aug;1172:34-53.

behavioral response. For example, if you've fallen behind in your loan payments, rather than panic, you decide to find a way to resolve the situation, such as getting a second job to support those payments. Or if you're told you have cancer and that it is treatable, rather than worry about dying, you focus on the surgery and recovery at hand. On the other hand, if you assess a situation and decide that there is nothing you can do to alter the course and just accept it or give in, you will begin a more cognitive or mind-based strategy that allows you to come to terms with the situation emotionally.

A landmark study by Dr. Elissa Epel and her colleagues provided a physiological theory on how we respond to stress.[137]

A positive emotional state gives a person a sense of well-being, balance, and self-control. This stimulates a hormonal response of testosterone and growth hormone, both important in the routine healing and repairing of the body. Notably, serotonin secretion also increases.[138]

In contrast, stress messes up the body's neuroendocrine system, resulting in a change in the diurnal (day–night) rhythm of cortisol secretion and elevating its baseline level. This, in turn, increases our insulin production, which we discussed in an earlier chapter. These combined actions lead to damaging effects in our bodies caused by glycation and oxidative stress.[139, 140, 141]

But how is it possible to accurately determine when a situation will be critically stressful enough to affect the biology of your body? When you "read" a stressful situation appropriately and use the proper coping strategy, your body secretes hormones that optimize your health. But if you evaluate a stressful situation in the opposite way (for example, you try to control an uncontrollable situation, like your risk of contracting COVID-19 while working in an ICU), your stress will not subside, and destructive hormones will be secreted. In other words, *perceived control* is a crucial indicator of stress resilience.

It's hard to predict who might be most vulnerable to chronic stress. Time will tell if frontline workers, especially in hospital ICUs, experience uncontrolled stressors. What we *can* do is try to improve our ability to interpret stressful situations correctly. Essentially, it's good to know when to fold your cards, when to ask for help, and when to fight. Because so many people would not and could not fold their cards, many people have sought mental health support. At the beginning of this chapter, we discussed the MetLife study. That study also found that 48% of employees sought help using an employer resource, a jump of 43% from the year prior.[142]

With the ongoing pandemic, we continue to deal with more stress than ever before. And even when we have regained some degree of new normal back into our lives, there will be new stressors to address – we will continue to experience the economic impacts of COVID-19, our children's academic learning will likely need some catch-up, and we will feel social pressures to find the time to reunite with family and friends in person.

So let's consider the healthy coping tools you can use to stay positive. You can start by channeling your negative emotions (such as fear, anxiety, and panic) into goal-oriented, meaningful plans. People are dealing with the pandemic in different ways. Some embrace the situation and find higher purpose and reasons for why COVID-19 has struck us. All of us have had to reflect on the importance of family and friends, our neighborhoods, and communities. Many have done a significant amount of volunteer work during this pandemic to give back and pay it forward. My team at the clinic took it upon ourselves to give back to the community – we raised funds and sourced personal protective equipment (PPE) to improve the safety of frontline health workers. It was our way to de-stress and it helped us cope.

My Masking Together Challenge

At the beginning of this book, I shared with you the emotional turmoil I experienced because I no longer worked in the hospital and was no longer part of the front line. I soon realized that I could still contribute to my community by leveraging the generosity and expertise of my clients and their companies to support my Masking Together Challenge.

With support from Dr. Trevor Young, Dean at the Faculty of Medicine, University of Toronto, we agreed that Canada's need went far beyond masks. Partnering with my alma mater, we set our goals to meet three challenges:

Here are our three challenges from the first campaign:

1. Find all types of personal protective equipment to fill the inventory gaps for our frontline health teams at all hospitals affiliated with University of Toronto.
2. Support our residents and fellows, who are specialists in training, to find a safe place to self-isolate. These individuals may pose risks to their families if they return home after working shifts to care for COVID-19 patients, or they may be simply too tired to drive home safely afterward.
3. Fund urgent research, going beyond the search for a COVID-19 vaccine. There is much more to learn and understand in how we can deploy countermeasures to reduce the spread of the virus.

All frontline workers providing various services during this COVID-19 pandemic are at three times higher risk for contracting COVID-19 – even with PPE. Vulnerable communities are far more likely to not only contract COVID-19, but also to die from it. Those who take care of them in our shelters and on the streets are the invisible front line.

For our invisible frontline workers and their clients, physical risks and mental health difficulties dramatically increase without access to medical-grade PPE and psychosocial supports to stay safe. Our community services and shelters are underfunded at the best of times, but as these communities' needs grew during this pandemic, their budgets did not.

In our second campaign, from December 2020 to the present, we focused on the invisible frontline healthcare workers who work in our communities to take care of the vulnerable living on the streets and in shelters. During this pandemic, community groups who manage homeless shelters, homes for abused women and their children, community centers, LGBTQ drop-in centers, and street youth hubs have all been forgotten. The workers and shelters did not receive any PPE from governments to keep them safe. To date, we have made direct donations of masks, face shields, hand sanitizers, and cleaning materials, totaling over $150,000 in value.

It is essential to recognize that all communities and neighborhoods need access to the supplies and supports required to squash this COVID-19 virus.

We are not safe until all of us are safe.

Faith

Another mind–body connection can be found in spiritual well-being. People who lead a "faith-based" life often live longer than those who don't. Perhaps it has something to do with a religious coping strategy – a faith that your life is manageable and in the hands of a higher power.[143, 144]

I'm not advocating that you should become religious. Rather, I'd suggest that we must all develop and practice a value system that fosters higher purpose, setting our goals beyond those that our materialistic society says are good for us – so that when adversity hits, we can attribute a meaning to it and discover a way to reason with the situation, and to control it. Certainly, for many of us, the material items we used to hold as necessary, such as fashionable clothing and makeup, have become irrelevant as we work from home and wear masks while outside during the pandemic lockdowns.

Meditation and other contemplative practices all promote a sense of direction and purpose in our lives. Our priorities shift away from self-gratification and hedonic experiences to more genuine contentment and a stronger sense that we contribute to and are part of our community. Many studies, including a growing number of happiness studies, support the idea that when we see life as meaningful, we automatically use more flexible coping strategies and have greater resilience around stress.[145]

Before the lockdowns, I was struck by a lecture I attended at the Rotman School of Management in Toronto, Canada. The venerable Tenzin Priyadarshi is the Dalai Lama Center for Ethics and Transformative Values at MIT in Boston and is a Tibetan Buddhist monk. He teaches the ethics and leadership program at MIT Sloan and other universities worldwide, including the Rotman School.

Priyadarshi asked the audience if they were happy. Then he told a short story about a man who picked him up from the airport in his new Bentley car. The man appeared very happy because of his new car and began describing its attributes. Suddenly, he saw another Bentley coming his way, and he noted it was a newer model with more upgrades. Suddenly he didn't appear to be so happy anymore.

Priyadarshi asked the audience, "What is happiness?" How do we find this place of low stress? He went on to note that many of us change our cars, homes, jobs, and even spouses (sometimes a few times) in an attempt to "find happiness" and to demonstrate our life's "successes." Yet we are not satisfied. Why not?

Many of us still measure our level of success in life through our net worth. I encourage you to measure it by your self-worth. To do so requires that you find a sense of life purpose, which will go a long way toward your longevity. Simply put, when you have no purpose in life, your mind and body begin to die.

If we can just "see" things differently or get out of stressful situations, our bodies will not be as damaged by our stress response as they would be if we did nothing. So the goal here is to thrive when you're being pummeled by adversity from this pandemic and its aftereffects. Find a higher purpose and develop a new sense of empowerment and control over the new challenges before you.

Pet Therapy

Many of us have pets, and most people smile widely when they meet a friendly dog or graceful cat. At the beginning of the first wave of the pandemic, pets were in short supply, along with many other things. Many people adopted pets from shelters. It certainly was a new distraction and an excuse to go outdoors for longer walks, but did it help people cope with life and reduce their stress at home?

There is a wide body of research now proving pets are good for your health and mental well-being. Most of the studies were done with dogs, often our best friend.[146]

Handlers have brought dogs into nursing and retirement homes to socialize with the elderly and disabled, to support healthy aging. Animal interactions improve life satisfaction and decrease depression in older adults, irrespective of whether they have dementia or other cognitive deficits.[147]

War veterans can also benefit from animal interactions. Another study showed that dogs and horses can reduce depression, post-traumatic stress disorder (PTSD) symptoms, and anxiety in war veterans with PTSD. Most studies were not vigorous, but they provided some evidence that this animal-assisted intervention, a treatment named by psychiatrists, has this potential.[148]

In other demographics, pet therapy can improve positive emotions, reduce negative emotions, and lower perceived stress in university students. Thousands of universities have created Pet Your Stress Away programs for students during stress-filled final examinations weeks.[149, 150, 151]

Finally, in 2019, a group of researchers at Washington State University confirmed that spending just 10 minutes with a cat or dog improved students' moods, but most importantly, they experienced stress-reducing physiological benefits by lowering their cortisol hormone levels.

Two hundred and fifty students were divided into four groups to compare the effects of different pet interaction experiences. Cortisol levels were checked upon waking in the morning and again before the test. Group 1 had hands-on interactions in small groups with the pets for 10 minutes. Group 2 first observed other people petting animals before getting access to them for 10 minutes. Group 3 only watched a slideshow of Group 1's interactions, while Group 4 didn't experience any pet interactions (they were the "waiting" control group).

Salivary cortisol samples collected after the pet interactions revealed that Group 1 showed significantly less cortisol in their saliva, followed by Group 2. It's interesting to note that Group 3's cortisol also lowered compared to Group 4, the control group.

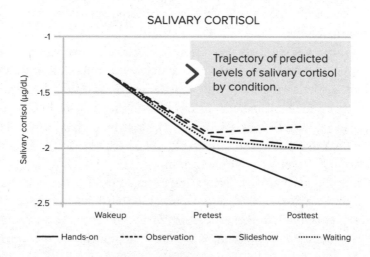

SALIVARY CORTISOL

Trajectory of predicted levels of salivary cortisol by condition.

Clearly, the study demonstrated that cortisol levels were lower than expected all around after the pet interactions, no matter if these interactions involved true touch or just a visual experience – which may suggest that visual experiences can be an important tool for reducing stress.[152]

Creative Arts Therapies (CATs)

Most would agree that all forms of art feel good for our soul, whether we experience it with our vision, hearing, touch, taste, or smell. But does it, in fact, support mental well-being? The answer is an empathic yes!

Major creative art forms include visual art, music, dance/movement, and drama. As forms of therapy, they all have shown in scientific studies to reduce stress and can be used as stress-management tools.[153]

So many of my clients decided to return to painting and sculpting during the lockdowns. They found it to be a great way to escape from the stress of the pandemic. Even my son signed up for a theater class at college to tap into his creative side and benefit from the social interaction, even though it was all virtual.

Psychologists use various words and phrases – such as *interception* to describe a body experience, *access emotions* to describe physical expression, and *embodied appraisal* to describe changed behavior – to explain why creative arts help reduce stress. This is all to say, creative arts are a way of physically expressing how we feel using verbal, nonverbal, and symbolic communication.

In art therapy, patients use different materials – like paint, crayons, and clay – to create two- and three-dimensional works to express their feelings. Artistic expression can also be explored in the kitchen too. During this pandemic, many of us have found time to cook in the kitchen again, and use takeout as a reprieve. During the early months of lockdown, flour and yeast were often sold out at grocery stores, as families decided to bake and make treats again.

I'm confident that we crave eating at restaurants because it's simply one of the ways to experience art – in a food format – where all of our senses are stimulated. Food looks so lovely on the table, and we take photos to share on Instagram. As we dive into a meal, we can smell the scents and taste the savory and sweetness. Certainly, finger foods provide another sensory stimulus. And finally, we have friends and family together, and we are inspired to share ideas that spark interest in new experiences and adventures.

From a more medical perspective, psychiatrists and psychologists use art to communicate with young children who may have difficulty in expressing how they feel after significant stress and trauma. Not only does the art become informational for the mental health specialist, but it's also therapeutic for the children because they can release their emotions.

Many people have created great pieces of art, using them as their emotional outlet. Pablo Picasso is well-known for his manic-depression tendencies, and one can only assume that art was his escape, or "treatment."[154]

There is no doubt that creating any artwork is an excellent physical activity that can help you cope with emotional angst.[155]

There is one universal language that brings the world together – music and its physical expression, dance. I can recall only a few times during this pandemic where I saw something that moved me to tears of joy: scenes where entire neighborhoods sang in unison on their balconies in Italy, opera and Broadway stars sang for passersby, neighbors banged their pots and pans each night in support of frontline workers, and kids line danced in the streets to encourage their neighbors to come out and dance.

Everyone has experienced how fast-paced music has the power to make us feel happy and generally more alert. Calmer and slower sounds relax our minds and allow us to better concentrate – case in point: my work environment as I write this book. Music is easy to access and freely available. Research studies confirm that music is an effective therapy for stress management.

We can encourage relaxation by choosing music that syncs with our alpha brainwaves, which are paced at 60 beats per minute. To get to sleep, our alpha waves must change to delta waves, which range from 2 to 3 cycles per second. To reach this state, you need to listen to calm music for about 45 minutes.[156] Imagine music as sleep medicine. It works!

Sound Baths

Check out these types of music, which help improve relaxation[157]:

- Native American
- Celtic
- Indian stringed instruments
- Jazz
- Classical (such as Dvorak's Symphony No. 9, the "Largo" movement)
- Easy listening and spa
- Soft and steady drums
- Nature sounds, such as rain and thunder

You can measure your brainwaves using a device called an electroencephalogram (EEG). One such device I use to relax and meditate with music or natural sounds is the Muse Headband, which provides me with a readout of my sessions and shows my brain frequencies. I can use it not just while awake, but also during sleep.

Music and dance therapy, as health professionals like to call it, is alive and thriving! It works by taking our minds off our stressors and effectively lowers our anxiety through physical and creative means.[158]

Ecotherapy

We just highlighted the benefits of listening to nature's sounds to lower stress. There is also a strong correlation between time spent in nature and reducing stress, anxiety, and depression. Many families have made an effort on weekends to hike together and get outside, even just in their neighborhoods. I have discovered so many things about my community simply because I made an effort to get outside, walking or running.

Bringing nature indoors, by way of plants and images of nature, can also make a difference. No one can dispute how good we feel with a vase of flowers in our home!

Being outdoors can lower your blood pressure and cortisol levels. Our prefrontal cortex is active during high stress and depression.

Rumination, or repetitive thoughts, increase, which can be detrimental to our mental health, especially if they are negative thoughts. It is a survival short circuit screaming, "Get out of here!" In other words, a fight-or-flight reaction in response to stress. Thankfully, being outside in nature appears to calm this reflex right down. Nature also increases our feel-good hormones (endorphins) and increases our dopamine, which leaves us feeling satisfied.[159, 160]

Having something to look at, even trees and nature, out your window can also be helpful. When the pandemic started, I turned my home and office desks to face a window. I have also made it a habit to have a plant near me. Orchids are great; they last for a few months and need little care.

Start making it a habit to get outdoors for at least 10 to 15 minutes each day – ideally up to 50 minutes to see some measurable positive physiological effects.

Cannabis Use

I'll close out this chapter by discussing the use of cannabis to relax and de-stress. The use of cannabis has increased during this pandemic, as we noted in Chapter 2, and this is no surprise.

In many parts of the world, including Canada and some states in America, the personal use and retail sale of cannabis has been decriminalized. There are many potential benefits of cannabis, but it is not a panacea to cure all that ails us. Some medical conditions have good supportive scientific evidence showing cannabis can improve symptoms, and other studies show promise.

Many cannabis components belong to a class of molecules known as cannabinoids; CBD (cannabidiol) and THC (tetrahydrocannabinol) are the two most abundant. Other cannabis components belong to a molecular class known as terpenes.

Cannabis sativa and cannabis indica are the two primary subspecies from which most commercial cannabis strains are derived. These subspecies tend to produce contrasting effects because sativa is enriched for THC whereas indica is enriched for CBD.

Hemp is a variety of cannabis that has low to zero THC and a high level of CBD. Hemp products, such as hemp oil and hemp-extracted CBD oil, have high CBD levels and low to zero THC.

Cannabis impacts the body's physiological functions through a cellular signaling pathway known as the endocannabinoid system (ECS). This system affects many biological processes, including metabolism, appetite, pain, sleep, mood, learning and memory, cardiovascular function, gastrointestinal function, the immune system, and neural development.

Terpenes are aromatic oils that color cannabis varieties with distinctive "flavors." Each terpene is associated with unique effects. Some terpenes promote relaxation and stress relief, while others promote focus and acuity.

Research studies have shown that cannabis can help with pain management and reduce seizure intensity and frequency. More studies are underway to demonstrate its usefulness in neurogenerative disorders, inflammatory bowel disease, and irritable bowel syndrome, and in the treatment of mental illnesses such as depression, anxiety, and post-traumatic stress syndrome (PTSD). Of interest to many who have insomnia is cannabis's impact on improved sleep.[161]

Few formal medical studies have been done to demonstrate the toxicity profile in medical cannabis users. To date, no significant adverse effects have been noted in countries that have legalized cannabis use.

Different strains of cannabinoids and terpenes are effective at treating various types of health conditions. A cannabis product that is good for one individual may not be suitable for another person because of variables such as genetics and individual medical conditions.

You can reduce any trial-and-error side effects by knowing your drug metabolism tendencies toward THC and CBD. A pharmacogenetics test will not only provide you and your prescriber with this valuable knowledge, but it will also show how cannabis might interact with any other drugs that you consume, including alcohol and caffeine. Genetic testing can also offer insights into cannabis efficacy in treating certain health conditions.

In the following section, let's focus on your recovery. We want a healthy body and mind that are resilient to unexpected illness and chronic health conditions. It's easy to say, "Eat well to be of ideal weight, get enough good-quality sleep regularly, and make sure you stay active and exercise daily." But what is the latest science on diets? How does one achieve sound sleep? What else can you do beyond getting on a treadmill to work out?

RECOVERING THE BODY AND MIND

CHAPTER 8

ACHIEVING HEALTHY WEIGHT

*Proven scientific strategies for eating well,
losing weight safely, and keeping it off*

CHAPTER 9

REST IS BEST

*Strategies to achieve the highest quantity
and quality of sleep*

CHAPTER 10

BEYOND BEING ACTIVE

*Benefiting fully from your workouts and
other forms of activities*

CHAPTER 8

Achieving Healthy Weight

Nature versus Nurture

Fifteen years ago, I first appeared on CNN to talk about the power of genetics. And The *Globe and Mail* interviewed me for a front-page story on New Year's Eve 2005 titled "Would You Gaze into a Genetics Crystal Ball?" about the new world of consumer genetics. At the time, many people were concerned they might inadvertently learn when they would die and from what causes. But even today we still can't discover this information, based on genetics.

Fast-forward to today and we as a society are generally more comfortable with the idea of genetics testing. There has been a surge in its use in personalized medicine, especially in the realm of diagnosing genetic disorders and treating cancer. North America makes up two-fifths of the market share of genetics testing globally, making it the largest adopter of genetics testing.

Genetics and COVID-19 Vaccines

Without modern science's ability to sequence genomes (a complete DNA reading), we would not have the ribonucleic acid (RNA) vaccines we now have to fight COVID-19. Thank goodness!

Some of the newest vaccines now in circulation are called messenger ribonucleic acid (mRNA) vaccines. Naturally occurring mRNAs are molecules in our cells that pass on genetic instructions from our DNA to make amino acids and then proteins, the building blocks of life. Each of us makes millions of copies of mRNA daily. These provide the directions to build everything necessary for life, including enzymes, hormones, muscle and nerve tissues, liver and skin cells, and everything you can think of that your body produces to allow for daily function and survival.

Manipulating mRNA molecules to fight disease has been a promising technology in the lab for more than 30 years. Pharmaceutical companies were already working to produce a vaccine platform using mRNA before the pandemic hit.[162] Thankfully, the technology was ready to build out a COVID-19 vaccine.

Some labs, such as BioNTech (who partnered with Pfizer to create the first mRNA COVID-19 vaccine), have been developing immune-suppressive treatments for cancer since 2017.[163]

Working with Regeneron, BioNTech was the first company, in June 2020, to successfully create an immunotherapy treatment for melanoma using RNA cancer vaccines, which stimulated the immune system to kill cancer cells.[164]

Unlike traditional vaccines, which are made using a portion of the real virus and often grown slowly in chicken eggs, these mRNA molecules can be produced rapidly in a lab, programmed with a bit of the coronavirus's genetic code for its spike proteins.

The COVID-19 vaccine contains mRNA. Once inside our body, the vaccine mRNA does what our natural mRNA does. With the help of other molecules, called ribosomes (think of them like the factory equipment), the mRNA produces a portion of the SARS-CoV-2 virus spike protein inside our body.

Once our body realizes this small portion of spike protein is an invader, the immune system creates antibodies to remove it from the body. If and when an actual SARS-CoV-2 virus attacks your body, the immune system quickly recognizes, attacks, and neutralizes it using the antibodies already "in storage," thanks to the vaccine. Therefore, think of the vaccine as a primer.

To be clear, the mRNA vaccine instructs your healthy cells to make many of the same pieces of spike protein. They can't make you sick, but they will teach your body's immune system what the virus looks like. Just as people had concerns many years ago about genetics testing, some ask me if the mRNA vaccines can alter their DNA. Absolutely not! The mRNA vaccines carry instructions to your body on how to build a protein, not build DNA. It does not go into your genetic material. RNA is a photocopy of a DNA code.

Personalized Medicine and Genetics

Genetics companies like 23andMe have offered consumer population genetics testing since 2006. This statistical calculation of your genetic risk is based on a group of naturally occurring genetic markers, or SNPs (single-nucleotide polymorphisms). These SNPs have been found to increase the risk of certain disease conditions, especially in diseases such as diabetes, Alzheimer's disease, macular degeneration (the leading cause of severe vision loss in people over 60), atrial fibrillation (a kind of cardiac arrhythmia), and certain types of cancer. Geneticists at these companies bundle a group of SNPs into a condition and provide a statistical estimate based on how many SNPs your DNA possesses. If you score higher than the average population, you should probably keep an eye on the condition and take steps to screen yourself more often. Presently I suggest patients revisit their genetics profile every few years and retest; a genetics panel becomes more accurate and precise as more research is done on certain SNPs.

Over the years, I've started to do targeted testing, which focuses on improving your lifestyle and especially your diet to guide you with clearer knowledge based on your genetics. This is the idea behind nutrigenomics, to eat according to your genetic profile. It's a scientific fact that we all respond differently to the foods and drinks we consume. With today's technology, you can determine the effect of salt on your blood pressure; whether you are lactose intolerant or a celiac; how well you can absorb certain nutrients, such as folic acid, vitamin C, and omega fatty acids from the food you consume; and even whether caffeine is "good" for you – a popular question! Some genetics reports outline what specific balance of carbohydrates, protein, and fat you should eat. I'm still not convinced of the precision of this, of following a diet based on genetics alone, given there are always nurture factors involved.

Scientists study identical twins to determine the roles that nature and nurture play in our development. You won't be surprised to learn that identical twins are born with the same genetics; where and how one twin grows up compared to the other can impact their overall health.

> "Genetics loads the gun but the environment pulls the trigger."[165]
> — *George Bray, American obesity researcher,*
> *Professor Emeritus Louisiana State University*

Nature versus Nurture

Many scientists agree that while there has been a steady rise in obesity over the last few decades, as we discussed in an earlier chapter, the skewing to severe obesity is disproportionate to those genetically at risk for obesity. Research suggests that those who have a higher genetic risk of obesity are more particularly susceptible to the modern lifestyle environment.[166]

Our genes impact how we crave and metabolize our food. We know that being in an environment that stimulates us to overeat, such as at a buffet, can cause those with a genetic predisposition to feel less full to eat more than they need. This leads to too many calories ingested and weight gain.[167]

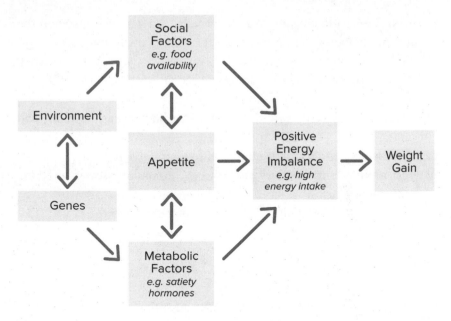

Adapted from Source: Reproduced from Llewellyn and Fildes

Food for Health

I've always said that food is our first-line "drug." Certainly, it is our first line of defense. No one can doubt anymore the straight-line link between what we eat and our health. While all of us want to consume foods that promote our health, we also want foods that match our lifestyle, culture, and genetics. But is there a perfect formula for what foods are best for you? Sorry, no. Why? Because your ideal diet may be different from mine. There's no one-size-fits-all solution when it comes to truly personalized nutrition.

So what's the key to finding the *right* healthy diet for you?

You can assess your biomarkers to know which facets of the aging processes are going on in your body and what nutrients you're deficient in. Only then can you modify your diet accordingly and, if need be, add a few key supplements to boost your overall health.

All of that said, I have noticed that my patients share a few pervasive diet problems. Perhaps you'll find them true for you too. Is the food on your dinner plate balanced nutritionally? Do you ever question the quality of the food you buy? Do you get tired or "crash" during the day? Could it be you're not getting the right nutrients? Or maybe you have a food sensitivity. Here are four patterns I see all the time.

1. Meals don't have the right balance of carbohydrates, proteins, and fats.
2. The quality and nutrient quality of food are questionable.
3. An unknown food allergy, sensitivity, or intolerance is affecting nutritional health.
4. We eat our meals at all times (and wrong times) of the day.

Getting Your Diet-Balancing Act Together

When you eat a balanced meal that contains all three sources of food fuels, you provide your body with all three kinds of energy, leading to a better total energy picture over a 5- to 6-hour period. Equally important, a balanced diet provides all the micronutrients (vitamins and minerals) that impact the strength of our immune system so it can fight infections. Your body converts carbohydrates, proteins, and fats into energy at different rates depending on your genetics.

FOOD FUELING

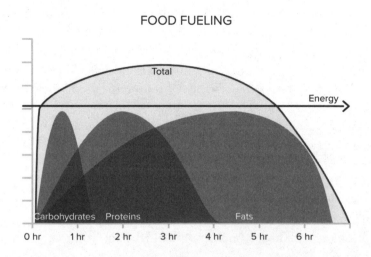

There are three types of food fuels.

1. Carbohydrates: These plant-based foods provide an almost instantaneous energy source in the form of sugars. The energy comes quickly, but it also fades quickly. Examples include grains (such as wheat, rice, oats), fruits, and vegetables.
2. Proteins: Proteins come from both plant and animal sources. They provide the same amount of caloric energy as carbohydrates but are not as readily available to your body. They provide an intermediate source of energy. Examples of plant sources are chickpeas and quinoa, and animal sources include meat (such as chicken, beef) and seafood (such as fish, shrimp).
3. Fats: All fats provide higher caloric energy than both carbohydrates and proteins from plant and animal sources. However, this food fuel supplies your body with energy hours after ingesting and digesting it and for a longer time. Examples of plant sources are cooking oils (such as olive, grapeseed, avocado), and animal sources include dairy (such as milk, cheese, butter) and fat attached to the meat.

What Secrets Your Teeth Reveal

Do you ever think that we were genetically designed to eat meat? The clue is in our teeth. Our eight premolars and 12 molars (including wisdom teeth) work to grind grains, seeds, vegetables, and fruits. Our eight incisors are there to help us bite and tear into foods. Note that we have only four canine teeth to cut meat. For this reason, I believe our mouths are sending us a message: we do need meat, just not that often.

Moderation is key. After all, when humans had to hunt for meat, they weren't always successful. It's not like the meat came right to them as it does for us today in the grocery aisle. People who live the longest (such as those in Japan, Sardinia, and Costa Rica) share a common trait: they don't eat anywhere near as much meat as the average North American does. When they do serve meat, it's usually on a special occasion.

Assuming you are generally healthy, of normal weight, and have no medical issues, conventional wisdom has been to break down your food group proportions into the following percentages:

Carbohydrates: 45%–65%
Proteins: 10%–35%
Fats: 20%–35%

Sound about right? Maybe. It all depends on your genetics, health, and lifestyle needs. It did sound good in the 1980s, but it turns out that conventional wisdom was wrong to overload on carbohydrates and to cut back fats.

In the early 1970s, researchers discovered the low-density lipoprotein (LDL), or "bad," cholesterol sub-particle and later found it to be high in dietary fats. Researchers also saw a correlation between LDL cholesterol and cardiovascular disease. So the logical conclusion was that dietary fats increased cardiovascular disease. Hence, the next step was to reduce the proportion of fats in our diets and substitute them with carbohydrate foods (such as bread and pasta) that were also lower in calories (4 kilo-calories per gram compared to 9 kilocalories per gram for fats).

The Heart and Stroke Foundation of Canada, the American Heart Association, the American Stroke Association, and many other medical associations endorsed these guidelines to decrease our fat intake from 40% to 30% and to boost our carbohydrate intake. They all believed that this was the correct way to lower cardiovascular disease. As a result, these guidelines became eating gospel for the next 30 years.

According to a report published by the Centers for Disease Control and Prevention, over a span of 3 decades (between 1971 and 2000), North Americans' diets changed drastically because the percentage of calories from fat they consumed decreased.[168] This sounds like good news. But it hasn't worked out that way. It turns out that the calories consumed rose by 22% in women and 7% in men over those same 30 years. For women, that is the equivalent of adding 335 calories to your diet every day – or a small Dairy Queen banana split.

How did this shift around cholesterol change the health of North Americans?

- As a society, we are now generally 25 pounds (11.5 kg) heavier than we were 25 years ago. Shocking!
- Heart disease has not dramatically decreased.
- Obesity and diabetes are at epidemic levels in North America.
- Children are rapidly becoming more obese than their parents, and many may even die of complications of diabetes (heart disease and stroke) *before* their parents die.

So it turns out that medicine got it wrong. To understand why, we need to look at the assumptions these decisions were based on. More than a few assumptions were sadly off the mark.

The first fallacy? That cholesterol is a direct contributor to heart disease. A correlation is not the same as causality. In other words, just because something's related doesn't mean that that relation involves cause and effect. The problem with the eating strategy in the 1980s was that no one had yet proven that LDL "caused" heart disease.

We were wrong when we started to think of and "treat" cholesterol as its own disease. Using statin (cholesterol-lowering) prescription medications seemed beneficial because they seemed to slow heart disease progression. This observation enhanced the theory that cholesterol caused heart disease. We now know more about what statins do: they may well be acting more effectively to slow down the rate of developing heart disease because of their anti-inflammatory and antioxidant effects.[169]

Statin Medications and COVID-19

During this past year, we've learned that a pro-inflammatory cholesterol derivative called cytokines causes much of the lung injury in COVID-19 cases of pneumonia. Recently it was discovered that those who had been taking statin medications had improved COVID-19 outcomes.

In fact, in 12 comparative studies, statin users reduced their mortality risk by 47% compared to non-statin medication users.

Statin medications are also known for their anti-inflammatory, plaque stabilization, and antithrombotic (anti-clotting) properties.[170]

Sugar: Not Sweet, But Toxic

The guidelines of the 1980s also suggested carbohydrates were better for us than fats. Many of us developed our sweet tooth and our love of breads and pasta during this time. And during the pandemic, we ate far more of it than we should have. Most of us know better. Sugar is a carbohydrate, and there's no doubt about it: sugar is bad for us. In fact, it's so bad that some doctors and scientists have declared a war against sugar. One such doctor is Dr. Robert Lustig, a pediatric endocrinologist at the University of California. He is one of the first in his field to take serious steps to address sugar overload in today's society. He's written several books on the topic, including *Fat Chance: Beating the Odds Against Sugar, Processed Food, Obesity, and Disease*. You'll want to check out his YouTube lecture "Sugar: The Bitter Truth."[171]

Our bodies are digesting more carbohydrates, or "sugars," than ever before. And not all carbohydrate calories are equal. Today, the sugars we ingest are not from natural sources, such as from fruit; instead, they come from processed and manufactured sugars and sugar substitutes. Although all carbohydrates break down into sugar within our bodies, they do so at different rates and in different ways depending on the source. Our pancreas and liver can't handle these man-made sugars as readily.

Finally, ingesting sugar is addictive.

In the late 1960s, a graduate student named Anthony Sclafani noticed that lab rats quickly ate up some Kellogg's Fruit Loops they accidentally discovered. He decided to design a test to measure their zeal for this sugary snack. Rats hate open spaces and prefer the corners of their cages. Sclafani put the Fruit Loops in the brightly lit open center of their cages, which they normally avoid. To his surprise, the rats overcame their instinctual fears and ran out into the open to gorge on the cereal.

Years later, in 1976, Sclafani was working on another study. He was trying to fatten some rats for an experiment but was unsuccessful when feeding them Purina Dog Chow. Recalling his observations years earlier, he decided to feed them sugar-laden products. The rats went crazy for the cookies and candies. They couldn't resist and became obese in just a few weeks. He published one of the first papers proving the incidence of food cravings.[172]

In the 2013 book *Salt, Sugar, Fat: How the Food Giants Hooked Us*, Pulitzer Prize–winner Michael Moss speaks about the food-industry term the *bliss point*. This point for sugar is the precise amount of sweetness or saltiness – no more, no less – that makes food and drink most enjoyable. At the Monell Chemical Senses Center in Philadelphia, scientists work to uncover the mechanisms of taste and smell and the psychology behind why we love certain foods so much. Moss interviewed scientists who conducted experiments to discover the bliss point of products for adults and children, as well as for geography and ethnic groups. The scientists discovered that children have a higher sugary bliss point than their parents. They also found that more African-Americans chose the sweetest and saltiest solutions than other ethnic groups.[173]

The truth gets even more bitter. Most of us recognize the obvious sugars, such as table (granulated) sugar, brown sugar, confectioners' (icing) sugar, honey, and corn syrup, plus the obvious sweetness found in sugary drinks and desserts. But I'm even more concerned about the hidden sugars found in so many processed foods, such as ketchup, barbecue sauces, and "fruit" yogurts – and even peanut butter. Some estimates claim that just 1 cup (250 mL) of peanut butter contains an average of 8 teaspoons (40 mL) of sugar!

Another big sugar source in our diets is the manufactured sweetener high-fructose corn syrup, which makes dietitians shudder. Although we are consuming less traditional sugar sourced from table sugar, we are consuming more high-fructose corn syrup because it is a cheaper alternative to sugar and is hidden in foods.

High-fructose corn syrup is included in so many foods because it helps foods taste smoother, compensating for the fats, such as butter, that we've removed from our carbohydrates. High-fructose corn syrup is found in almost everything shelved on the grocery store's inner aisles – soda, candies, jams, ketchups, and dressings. But more surprisingly, it is also found in some common "healthy" foods, such as yogurt, whole wheat bread, cereals, roasted nuts, and applesauce.

Our bodies love fructose because it is a naturally occurring form of sugar traditionally found in fruit, which also contains fiber. However, with man-made high-fructose corn syrup, we can obtain this sugar cheaply and in large amounts. But because it doesn't contain fiber, it is absorbed by our bodies at a faster rate. This speeds up the rate of blood sugar in the bloodstream, setting off an insulin response. The pancreas secretes more insulin to cope with the sudden sugar load. If you don't burn the sugar, you store it – as fat. And here you were, trying to avoid gaining weight as fat!

According to the United States Department of Agriculture, the average U.S. consumption of this man-made product dramatically increased from 8 ounces (250 g) in 1970 to 62.5 pounds (28.3 kg) per person in 2000. The good news? An increase in public health advocacy and a change in consumer habits have helped the overall consumption drop by half since then, to 36.7 pounds (16.6 kg) in 1 decade (2010). However, overall, North America continues to consume too much sugar and high-fructose corn syrup.

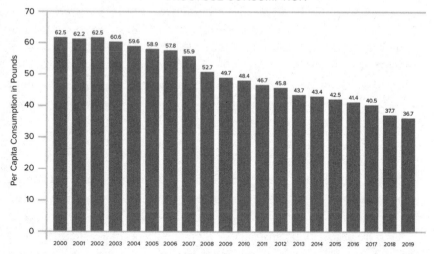

FRUCTOSE CONSUMPTION

Source: US Department of Agriculture; Economic Research Service ©Statista 2020

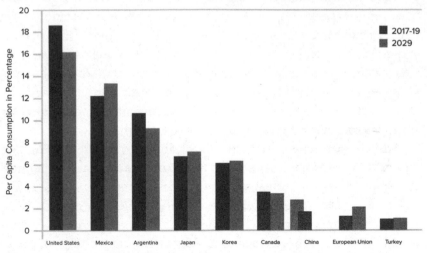

SWEETENER CONSUMPTION (COUNTRIES)

Source: US OECD/FAO (2020), "OECD-FAO Agricultural Outlook", OECD Agriculture statistics (database)

What Man-Made Sugars Do to Us

Studies done in 2011 by Dr. Kimber Stanhope, a nutritional biologist at the University of California, show that our livers process man-made sugars differently than natural sugars. In one study, participants consumed a normal low-sugar diet for a number of days; blood levels were taken to determine a baseline. The next portion of the study involved swapping out 25% of their calories for sweetened drinks containing high-fructose corn syrup. Participants' blood levels were tested every 30 minutes around the clock. At the end of the modified diet 2 weeks later, participants showed increased levels of LDL ("bad") cholesterol and other risk factors for cardiovascular disease.[174]

This study shows us that when we consume too much high-fructose sugar that is man-made, our livers become overloaded and convert a portion of it to fat as triglycerides, and fatty liver is the result.

How about Sugar Substitutes?

In July 2013, Susan Swithers, a behavioral neuroscientist at Purdue University, took aim at diet beverages and the reputation their manufacturers promote as healthy drink alternatives. In her mission, she scrutinized the most recent research on high-intensity sweeteners. She wanted to show that, despite the sweeteners' low-calorie contents, these drinks could cause a host of other health problems in those who consume them, such as weight gain and overeating. She focused on drinks that contain aspartame, sucralose, and saccharin (approximately 30% of American adults regularly consume these sweeteners in their diets). Following these evaluations, she suggested that diet soda may actually be as unhealthy as non-diet soda.

Artificial sweeteners affect the body's ability to track calorie intake and caloric needs. In other words, when the mouth tastes something sweet, the digestive system expects to receive calories and fat. Still, when these things never materialize, it confuses the body's metabolism. People feel hungry again, which causes them to eat more than they would if they'd consumed foods containing natural sugars. This response is known as the cephalic phase insulin release and it is triggered not only by our sense of taste but also by our senses of sight and smell. As well, in response to the sweetness of artificial sweeteners, the pancreas mistakenly thinks the sweet taste is real dietary sugar. Over time, chronically high insulin levels in the blood lead to decreased insulin receptor response, known as insulin resistance, a precursor to prediabetes and diabetes.[175]

The San Antonio Heart Study reported that artificially sweetened beverages also increased body weight in adults and teenagers compared to the same demographics who consumed beverages that had been sweetened with traditional sugar. And a host of other studies, including the Nurses' Health Study and the Health Professionals Follow-Up Study, reported greater risks for type 2 diabetes, heart disease, high blood pressure, and metabolic syndrome (a combination of disorders that, when occurring together, increase the risk of diabetes and cardiovascular disease) in people who consumed artificially sweetened beverages.[176, 177]

It's not difficult to imagine that people feel they can splurge in one area if they have saved in another on a psychological level. As some researchers call it, this cognitive distortion translates into consumers indulging in fat-heavy foods because they feel they are entitled to enjoy it – having just consumed fewer calories in their beverage. Some people call this the Diet Coke and French fries phenomenon.

Proteins and Veganism

Sometimes when we try to do something good for our health, and more recently for our environment, we unknowingly deprive ourselves of the nutrients our bodies really need.

A developing trend is the idea of becoming vegan (a form of vegetarianism that eliminates all forms of animal products from the diet). Although vegetarianism is common in many parts of the world, the key to following this diet correctly is to avoid potential pitfalls. Lowering fat intake, losing weight, or avoiding animal products for religious or ethical reasons can translate into a drop in protein intake. This results in nutrient and hormone deficiencies. But we all need protein, because our bodies convert it into three essential substances: enzymes, new proteins to be stored as muscle, and hormones – and none of us can function without these three things.

So what are the important components of proteins? Amino acids – the building blocks – are classified as essential amino acids (required for our bodies from our diet) and nonessential amino acids (ones that our bodies can manufacture from other amino acids). It's possible to obtain all of the eight essential amino acids from traditional types of animal proteins, but vegetarians will find this task more challenging because those amino acids aren't as easily tapped into by eating vegetables and legumes. Quinoa is on the rise as a popular vegetarian grain for this very reason: it is the only one that contains all eight essential amino acids.

Legumes, such as peas, peanuts, and beans, are alternative sources of nonanimal protein.

Low-Fat, Bad Fat, Good Fat, Fish Fat

Obesity rates have doubled since the 1980s, which was when we saw the first low-fat foods lined up on grocery shelves. In a weight-loss-crazed world, we've tried low-carbohydrate diets, low-fat diets, no-meat diets, all-protein diets, and everything in between, all to push our body to change its metabolism and shed pounds.

These diets emerged because saturated fats and trans fats had been deemed "bad" and it was believed they raise cholesterol levels and increase the risk for heart disease. Many fat-free foods are packed with sugar, refined carbohydrates, and calories to make them taste good. But just because a package says it's fat-free does not mean you can eat all you want. Tread carefully because the term *fat-free* can be a dieter's nightmare. Low-fat yogurt is a good example; you could forfeit fat and gain sugar. Eating Greek yogurt may be a smarter choice. It contains roughly half the carbohydrates of the regular kind of yogurt (5 to 8 g per serving compared to 13 to 15 g).

The low-fat diet also caused another problem: the dramatic decrease in essential, or "good," fats. These are known as monounsaturated fats and polyunsaturated fats, and they lower cholesterol, cut the risk of heart disease, and reduce inflammation.

Another group of important healthy fats is essential fatty acids (EFAs). Like essential amino acids, these fats cannot be synthesized by our bodies. They are necessary for biological processes but do not include the fats that we ingest or metabolize from our own fat stores into energy fuel.

The data consistently shows that most North Americans' diets are deficient in omega-3 fatty acids, comprised of eicosapentaenoic acid (EPA) and docosahexaenoic acid (DHA). These nutrients are essential for optimal brain and body health.[178]

We often eat the wrong types of fats, the fats found in fried foods and in red meats, which are inflammatory rather than anti-inflammatory.

Sources of Omega-3 Fatty Acids

The richest sources of essential fatty acids are oily fish, such as mackerel, herring, salmon, trout, and sardines. Strict vegetarians and vegans are more likely than meat-eaters to have low levels of EPA but also DHA. This is because foods such as nuts, seeds, dark leafy greens, and whole grains contain as little as 1% of the DHA that oily fish contain, and the only DHA-rich vegetable source is algae. (It's important not to consume too many large fish, such as red tuna, shark, or swordfish, because they contain high levels of mercury.)

Rarely do I hear of a family eating fish regularly. All too often, parents eat very little, and children eat none. Fish fats contain polyunsaturated fatty acids (PUFAs), or omega-3 and omega-6 fats, which break down into docosahexaenoic acid (DHA) and eicosapentaenoic acid (EPA). These critical nutrients are often found in very low amounts when I measure them in my patients. Only the people who eat fatty fish at least three times a week seem to have enough DHA and EPA in their bloodstream.

These acids can also be found in plants but in a different form of omega-3 called alpha linolenic acid (ALA). Seeds and seed oils – like flax, chia, and hemp – are especially rich in ALA. Other high-PUFA foods include nuts and avocados. The main problem with ALA is that it must be converted into EPA and DHA to exert the good effects attributed to omega-3s, and in plant-based foods, only about 11% of ALA is converted into EPA and DHA. In fish, the EPA and DHA are already present, so no conversion is needed. In other words, go ahead and add some flaxseed oil to your salad dressing, but know that it's not a substitute for the omega-3s in fish.

One benefit of omega-6 fatty acids is that they can prolong the shelf life of processed foods. And we need these fatty acids: they are integral to our nutritional health because they play a role in controlling how our cell membranes work. But these fatty acids must be properly balanced by omega-3 fatty acids to work well. And the bad news is that we don't consume enough omega-3s to reach this balance. In fact, the ideal ratio of omega-6 to omega-3 is 3:1 – yet the North American diet scores a balance between 15:1 and as high as 30:1. We eat far too few omega-3s and far too many omega-6s.

When we consume too many omega-6s, our cell membranes produce chemicals called cytokines, a direct cause of inflammation. You'll recall that cytokine-induced inflammation causes much of the lung injury in COVID-19 cases of pneumonia, so it's essential, especially now, to get the proper balance of omega-3 and omega-6 fatty acids in your diet.

Association Between Fish Consumption and Brain Health

We need adequate levels of DHA in our blood. Why? DHA deficiency is connected with a decline in how well our brains function, and it's been linked to degenerative conditions such as Alzheimer's disease. In other words, this could be a big concern as we age. One mechanism connected to this decline may be phosphatidylserine (PS). This is a phospholipid component that controls the auto cell death of weakening cells. What does this mean? Low DHA levels lower our neural cell PS level and quicken our neural cell death. As well, low levels of DHA are found in severely depressed people. Could low PUFAs be causing the increase of mental health problems in our society today? Perhaps.

A study found that, in women, each additional weekly serving of fish eaten decreased the risk of having a new bout of depression by 6%. And those who ate fish two or more times per week had a 25% lower risk of depression than those who ate less per week.[179]

Emerging clinical experience has demonstrated how an aggressive intake of omega-3 fatty acids is beneficial for patients with traumatic brain injury, concussion, and post-concussion syndrome. EPA and DHA help protect brain cells from oxidative stress. The brain needs to be saturated with high doses of omega-3 to heal.[180]

It's no surprise, then, that studies have also shown that 2 months' supplementation with 1 g of omega-3 fatty acids significantly reduces both the frequency and duration of migraines by 74%[181] – an improvement I have seen firsthand in my practice.

The Salt of the Earth

The phrase *salt of the earth* comes from the Bible, Matthew 5:13. "Ye are the salt of the earth: but if the salt has lost his savour, wherewith shall it be salted? It is thenceforth good for nothing, but to be cast out, and to be trodden under foot of men."

This idiom is used to describe people of great worth and reliability. It seems that the *salt of the earth* was a phrase coined about the value of salt at the time.

These days, salt has a bad rap. But salt, in itself, isn't a bad thing; it's the amount of salt we consume that is detrimental to our health. Our body can't produce salt on its own. Yet it requires this crystalline compound for several essential functions: to control our blood pressure, to transmit information between our cells in nerves and muscles, and to absorb nutrients from the small intestines during digestion.

Most of us don't realize that we're consuming too much salt. North Americans ingest about 3400 mg of salt per day. But health guidelines recommend we take in less than 2300 mg. This is equal to a single teaspoon of salt.

According to the Federal Drug Administration, 75% of the dietary sodium we consume comes from packaged and restaurant foods, not from the salt shaker. Some of the biggest culprits include cheese, processed meats (especially bacon), tomato sauce, salted cod and mackerel, anchovies, baked and refried beans, canned legumes, breads and rolls, and, of course, the salty condiments (like soy and teriyaki sauces).

When we consume too much salt, it throws off our body's fluid balance, and the body tries to bring levels back into proper balance by secreting the excess sodium. This essentially dehydrates the body and increases a hormone called angiotensin, which tends to increase blood pressure. And high blood pressure is a major risk factor for stroke, heart disease, and kidney disease. So it's important to always read the food labels to count your salt intake.

The Beauty of Water

Do you take a shower or bath every day? Or use moisturizers on your face? We wash our bodies with water and we lotion our skin, yet many of us forget the importance of water for the inside of our bodies. Everybody is different, and so is each body's water requirements.

The amount of exercise and activities you do, where you live, and your gender and age all affect your hydration needs. But despite the varying requirements of different people, everyone needs water.

Water makes up 60% of our body weight. And because our bodies are constantly losing water (through aspiration, perspiration, and urine and bowel movements, among other functions), we need to replenish that water by drinking more of it.

In fact, water is important to every one of our body's essential functions. It carries nutrients to your body's cells; aids in digestion; acts as a lubricant for mouth, nose, and ear tissues; improves skin tone and healthy muscles; flushes toxins from the body; helps the body fight bacteria and viruses that lead to inflammation and oxidative stress; and much more.

Different health organizations recommend varying amounts of water consumption. One of the most cited recommendations is from the Institute of Medicine in 2004, which suggests that men should drink 3.7 liters (13 cups) of total beverages every day, and women should drink 2.7 liters (9 cups).[182]

Beverages do not include caffeinated and alcoholic drinks because they dehydrate you. In fact, you should drink additional water when you consume such beverages. Food can also contribute to your hydration levels. According to the Mayo Clinic, food provides approximately 20% of a person's total water intake.[183]

If you're not sure if you're drinking enough water, pay attention to the color of your urine. The more yellow it is, the more dehydrated you are. Urine should be colorless or light yellow. Sip water throughout the day to stay hydrated – rather than drinking the recommended amount all at once.

Other factors can influence the color of your urine too, including some foods (beets and blackberries, for example), certain medications, and some vitamins (such as the B vitamin spectrum). Speak with your health professional if your urine is too dark.

Buyer Beware: Today's Hot Diet Is Tomorrow's Regret

The sheer number of trendy diets out there is overwhelming. Each one lures in a group of believers, who post over social media about how wonderful they feel after giving up something or doing just one thing. But which one of these diets can really help you lose weight and, more importantly, which ones are safe? Fad weight-loss diets are not something I would ever recommend. We must learn as a society to change our eating habits. One study, published in *American Psychologist* in 2007, merged the results of 31 earlier dieting studies and came to the frightening conclusion that, if anything, dieting is often a predictor of future weight *gain*. In fact, the study showed that up to two-thirds of dieters end up gaining more weight than they lost in the first place.[184]

Food Sensitivities that Restrict Our Diets

We all have a friend or family member who limits their diet in some way due to a food sensitivity. Of the many sensitivities – for example, lactose, preservatives, and additives – gluten is one of the most common. In 2012, gastroenterologists finally agreed that gluten sensitivity is a diagnosis separate from conditions such as celiac disease and wheat allergy. The criteria for diagnosing gluten sensitivity go beyond the usual spectrum of gastrointestinal symptoms. Checking for elevated levels of immunoglobulin G (IgG) and immunoglobulin A (IgA) – antibodies to a gluten protein called gliadin – can also help diagnose the problem.

DASH Diet

I want to introduce you to one diet. It is not a fad but based on sound science and reasonable parameters. The Heart and Stroke Foundation of Canada recommends this diet, and so do I. The basis of the diet is that we must begin by lowering dietary salt. The DASH diet, which stands for "Dietary Approaches to Stop Hypertension," is designed to lower blood pressure and support weight loss by reducing sodium (or salt) intake. High blood pressure and being overweight are known risk factors for many health conditions and, as you recall, a preexisting condition for higher risk of developing more severe COVID-19 illness.

As we discussed in Chapter 3, low-risk blood pressure is 120/80 mm Hg or less. Hypertension affects almost one in four adults, and the lifetime incidence of developing high blood pressure is estimated to be 90%.

The DASH diet has been shown to lower blood pressure in as little as 2 weeks. And the bonus is that it lowers LDL ("bad") cholesterol too. This diet has also helped many people lose weight over time.

We need salt, but not as much as you think. The DASH diet allows only 1500 mg of sodium per day, which is about two-thirds of a teaspoon. Compare this to an average intake of at least 3000 mg in most North Americans' diets.

The DASH diet emphasizes fruits, vegetables, whole grains, and low-fat or nonfat dairy, and it limits saturated fats and dietary cholesterol – a list of eating recommendations that sound like music to my ears.

Learn more at https://www.nhlbi.nih.gov/health-topics/dash-eating-plan.

Finally, let's summarize my three simple principles of healthy eating:

1. **Avoid refined grains and sugars.** Choose fruits, vegetables, beans, lentils, whole grains, lean proteins, and healthy fats.
2. **Burn fat between meals.** Never snack during the day, and exercise in the afternoon.
3. **Consider daily light eating – a form of intermittent fasting.** Try to eat your biggest meal in the morning and give yourself a window of 8 hours to eat. Avoid late-night eating.

How Is Caloric Restriction Different than Intermittent Fasting?

Healthy caloric restriction refers to ingesting foods with the highest nutritional value in the fewest calories possible, without the deprivation of essential nutrients, and is based on your activity levels. (It is not the same thing as dieting or enduring starvation.)

In contrast, an intermittent fasting diet requires a person to abstain from eating or to severely limit their intake during prescribed times of the day, week, or month. The result is a reduction in the overall number of calories consumed. During the holy month of Ramadan, Muslims are required to abstain from food and drink from dawn to dusk for 30 days.

We read about the benefits of maintaining nutritious, healthy eating habits and the health risks of doing the opposite. And research has also shown us that restricting calories can extend lifespan – at least with mice. In these animal studies, mice lifespans increased from 41 months to 56 months (120 to 150 human years) by following calorie-restricted diets.[185] Scientists believe that calorie restriction may increase our lifespan by increasing the levels of growth hormone.

To determine if the benefits of a restricted-calorie diet could also extend the lifespan of humans, scientists conducted a fascinating experiment in the early 1990s at a science research facility called Biosphere 2 in Arizona. For 2 years, scientists lived inside an air-locked structure where they cultivated and raised their own food sources. The foods they consumed were nutrient-rich, but they consumed 30% fewer calories than the average moderately active American male – about 2,500 calories per day.

At the end of the 2-year period, doctors evaluated the health of the Biospherians and found that they had lower cholesterol, blood pressure, and fasting blood sugar levels than when they entered the facility. Even after the scientists returned to their "normal" lives and went back to consuming foods as they did before the study, these levels remained low.[186]

I would be remiss if I didn't address the intermittent fasting trend. I have given my patients the green light to try this approach. The research suggests that this type of fasting causes a change in eating and sleeping patterns and, therefore, alters a person's metabolic rhythm. Most studies on the effects of Ramadan fasting do not demonstrate much weight loss but do show an increase in fat oxidation and a decrease in carbohydrate oxidation, resulting in lower insulin levels and improved cholesterol and blood sugar profiles.[187]

Some people who do intermittent fasting claim their memory and brain function improve. This is likely caused by the brain using ketones versus glucose to power up its cells. During fasting, the body first uses up glucose and glycogen (stored in our liver) to produce energy. After that, it uses fat. This type of stored energy is released from the fat in the form of ketones. Some researchers hypothesize that ketones are a more efficient energy source than glucose and may have antiaging effects on the brain.

However, it has been well documented that high ketone levels can also be harmful. In type 1 insulin-dependent diabetics, a condition known as ketosis can occur when blood sugars are too high.[188] The jury is still out on this type of lifestyle diet, but I can't stop anyone from trying it these days.

The Keto Diet

When people go on a strict keto diet, it generally prescribes 80% fat, 15% protein, and only 5% of carbohydrates. That translates into fewer than 100 calories a day from carbohydrates, including healthy ones like fruits and vegetables. When you eat this way, it triggers ketosis, which means your body begins to burn fat for energy, since it has burned through all its carbs as glucose or glycogen stores. We already know that burning too much fat, especially saturated fats, increases all the factors leading to coronary artery disease and inflammation.

Some people who follow the keto diet experience side effects. Symptoms of the keto flu include headaches, fatigue, muscle aches, breath that smells like nail polish remover (acetone), nausea, and diarrhea followed by constipation.

Circadian Rhythm Diet

Our bodies function best when we align our eating patterns with our circadian rhythms. Studies show that we should be eating only during daylight hours. This is a good place to begin if trying intermittent fasting to lose weight. I would strongly recommend that you read Dr. Satchin Panda's book titled *The Circadian Code*.[189]

I can certainly resonate with his belief that we were all shift workers before the pandemic, negatively impacting our health. A shift worker is defined as someone who stays awake for more than 3 hours between 10:00 p.m. and 5:00 a.m. for more than 50 days a year. We might not think of ourselves as shift workers, but rather as jet-lagged, late-night workers with parent duties and who get to bed late and get up early – and who've been doing so for far too many years. Of all the things that have positively impacted my C-suite patients, their lack of travel during the pandemic has had the biggest impact. Their overall health has improved. They have had to learn to stay at home, eat regularly, sleep in a regular bed, and interact with their spouse and kids. Novel life!

In my perfect world, we all follow our circadian rhythms. Every cell is our body has its own clock. In the morning, our body temperature, blood pressure, heart rate, and breathing rate all rise, and we have a higher metabolic rate. This is the best time to eat your biggest meal, and most of your carbohydrates should be eaten before 9 a.m. You should eat all the food you need for the day within an 8-hour window, according to a new study.[190] Following this eating pattern shows comparable weight loss to some conventional diets.

In the later afternoon, our muscle tone peaks, making it a good time to work out! By the evening, your body temperature begins to drop and your metabolism slows down. Therefore, later meals should be avoided. Research shows that eating late causes you to store more calories compared to eating in the morning.[191]

By sundown, the pineal gland begins producing melatonin, cortisol levels drop, and we get sleepy as the evening progresses. During sleep, the brain actively consolidates memories, flushes out toxins, and creates new neural connections.

"Eat breakfast like a king, lunch like a prince, and dinner like a pauper."[192]
— *Adelle Davis, American author, advocate for improved health through better nutrition, and considered the most famous nutritionist in the early- to mid-20th century*

Chinese Philosophy on the Body's Rhythm

Traditional Chinese medicine practitioners believe our body's energy runs in parallel with the sun and suggest the following schedule:

- 7 to 9 a.m.: Focus on the stomach; consume your biggest meal of the day.
- 9 to 11 a.m.: Focus on the pancreas and spleen.
- 11 a.m. to 1 p.m.: Focus on the heart.
- 5 to 7 p.m.: Focus on the kidney; consume a light dinner.

According to Dr. Panda, one single night of shift work can impact your memory and attention for a whole week. It will also cause a shift in appetite and the types of foods you crave. Certainly, all of us as doctors-in-training will recall our overnight shifts where we had sugar cravings and shared donuts and cakes with our nursing colleagues. Over time, these types of sleeping and eating behaviors increase obesity.

Earlier, we described the metabolic interaction between cortisol and insulin. In Chapter 9, I'll explain the metabolic impact of poor sleep.

CHAPTER 9

Rest Is Best

COVID Dreams

Earlier in the book, I shared the bizarre and frightening dreams that woke me up in the early months of the pandemic. I classified them as an extension of my PTSD, which I experienced during and after SARS, but these new dreams could easily be what many experience as simply COVID dreams. It turns out that I was not alone when I had my many vivid "pandemic dreams." The pandemic has not only interfered with our waking hours, it's also altered our dream world.

Thanks to social media, researchers were able to glean an unprecedented amount of data about dreams. Elizaveta Solomonova and Rébecca Robillard from the University of Ottawa, Canada, found that 37% of people aged 12 and older dreamed of being unable to complete tasks and being threatened by others.[193]

Other research showed people experienced emotional feelings of anger, sadness, and anxiousness, and felt stress in their dreams. Almost half of 100 nurses who treated COVID-19 patients in Wuhan, China, experienced nightmares – twice the lifetime rate among Chinese psychiatric outpatients and many times higher than the 5% of the general population who have nightmare disorders.

Much has now been published about people's curiosity related to the increase of their dreams in general, and vivid dreams and nightmares in particular, during the pandemic. Sleep scientists believe this is occurring because we are spending more time in bed and therefore experiencing more REM sleep.

Pandemic data confirms this increase in sleep time. The Chinese reported 34 minutes more sleep, while 54% of Finnish people said they slept more. In the United States, from March 13 to 27, 2020, there was a 20% increase in sleep time, especially in Maryland and New Jersey, where many residents have been spared a long daily commute to work.[194]

Researcher Bulkeley's 3-day research poll revealed that, in March 2020, 29% of Americans recalled more dreams than usual. Solomonova and Robillard found that 37% of people had pandemic dreams, many marked by themes of insufficiently completing tasks (such as losing control of a vehicle) and being threatened by others.

The Benefits of a Good Night's Sleep

Sleep is something we take for granted, and you may not realize how critically important it is for your good health. Although the role of sleep is complex, it's central to your survival and health, both in the short and long term. Here are just a few benefits of getting enough sleep:

- Sleep is critical for hormonal balance.
- Sleep is restorative for wound healing and immune system functioning.
- Sleep is needed for growth and rejuvenation in all of our body systems.
- Sleep affects brain development and brain normalcy later in life and is important for memory and mental processing.

However, many people do not get enough sleep. No doubt there are many reasons for this, including our work and home lives. As you'll learn later in the chapter, parents and people with certain types of jobs and health conditions suffer more from sleep deprivation or insomnia than others. Furthermore, the COVID pandemic has altered many people's sleep patterns.

COVID-Somnia

Since the onset of COVID-19, sleep disorder issues have risen along with other mental health issues. New schedules forced us to reset both our physical and biological clocks. Being in lockdown has meant less outdoor time and fewer chances to exercise, and these lifestyle changes continue on. Most cases of insomnia have been linked to the stressors caused by uncertainty and outright fear about COVID-19.

It's obvious that insomnia has become a pandemic concern: the word *insomnia* was googled 58% more times in 2020 (2.77 million times) than in each of the past 3 years.

At the University of Southampton, researchers found that the incidence of insomnia in their community increased from 1 in 6 people to 1 in 4 people. Not surprisingly, insomnia affected mothers, essential workers, and minority ethnic groups disproportionally. Key predictors were households with young children and perceived financial difficulties.[195]

During the first pandemic wave in China, insomnia rates rose to 20.0% from 14.6%, and in Greece in May 2020, 37% of respondents in a survey expressed they had insomnia.[196, 197]

One study in India researched the effects of pandemic sleep and discovered that not only have sleep schedules been altered, but night owls are affected more than early birds. Night owls tended to delay their bedtimes and waking times and slept fewer hours than the early birds who showed minimal sleep pattern changes. Daytime napping also increased, perhaps to overcome fatigue from sleep deprivation.[198]

Acute insomnia that is triggered by a sudden traumatic event, such as the sudden death of a family member, the loss of a job, and even an abrupt change in lifestyle during the early days of the pandemic, does not usually lead to a chronic sleep issue. However, about 1 in 5 cases of short-term insomnia do transition to chronic insomnia – which can persist in 40% to 70% of patients and for as long as 4 years.[199, 200]

As the pandemic continues to permeate our daily lives at home, work, and school, our sleep will continue to suffer and could lead to potential longer-term health and workplace productivity issues.

Sleep Deprivation Is a Global Crisis

Over a decade ago, scientists sounded the alarm at the World Health Organization and the Centers for Disease Control and Prevention (CDC). They called it a global epidemic of sleeplessness.

The American Academy of Sleep Medicine (AASM) and the National Sleep Foundation (NSF) recommend 7 to 8 hours of sleep for adults and 10 hours for school-age children.[201]

However, much of the population has been sleeping far less than these recommended guidelines – even before the pandemic. Studies show that nearly 40% of adults sleep an average of only 5 to 6 hours or less per night, while 69% of high school students sleep less than 8 hours on an average school night.[202]

A pre-pandemic annual survey of 2,000 people in the United States found that the average night's sleep decreased to 5 hours and 30 minutes in 2019 – from 6 hours and 17 minutes in 2018.[203]

A study of Norway high school students showed that 10% of them had developed "behaviorally induced insufficient sleep syndrome," a medical jargon way of saying these children chose to disregard good bedtime routines.[204]

Another study showed that sleep duration and daytime sleepiness vary by gender and marital status; women are more affected than men. Having children in a family unit also contributes to insufficient sleep among adults in the home.[205]

Around the world, insufficient sleep as a public health hazard has been ignored and underreported, and it has high economic costs.

Insomnia, directly and indirectly, costs the U.S. healthcare system $100 billion annually. The annual loss of quality-adjusted life-years from insomnia is far greater than the loss from other medical and psychiatric conditions, such as arthritis, depression, and hypertension.[206, 207]

There's no doubt that future studies will show an increase in the cost and pervasiveness of insomnia during and following the pandemic.

Lack of sleep not only costs us money and reduces our quality of life, it also increases our risk of premature mortality. A research work review showed that individuals who sleep for less than 6 hours per night had a ten-fold greater risk of premature mortality than those who slept 7 to 9 hours.[208]

People say, "Ah, I'll sleep when I'm dead." Well, an earlier death might occur faster than you think if you go without sufficient restorative sleep during your awake years.

Are You Sleep-Deprived?

Are you getting enough sleep? The common-sense way of figuring out that answer is to think about how you feel during the day. If you're getting enough sleep, you should be energetic and alert throughout your day. And it's not good enough to simply get enough sleep. If you're a poor sleeper, you could be missing out on the sleep cycles that are vital for the body and mind. It's not just quantity of sleep – sleep quality matters too.

Sleep Deprivation Symptoms

You might be sleep-deprived if you:

- Need an alarm clock to wake up on time
- Rely on the snooze button
- Have a hard time getting out of bed in the morning
- Feel sluggish in the afternoon
- Get sleepy in meetings, lectures, or on the bus/train
- Feel drowsy after heavy meals or when driving
- Need a nap to get through the day
- Fall asleep while watching TV or relaxing in the evening
- Feel the need to sleep in on weekends
- Fall asleep within 5 minutes of going to bed

Source: The National Institutes of Health.[209]

Insufficient Sleep "Syndrome"

Insufficient sleep is so serious that public health experts like to refer to it as a non-communicable disease.[210]

Definition: Insufficient Sleep

The International Classification of Sleep Disorders (ICSD-3) defines insufficient sleep as "a curtailed sleep pattern that has persisted for at least 3 months for most days of the week, along with complaints of sleepiness during the day. Further, a resolution of sleepiness complaints is shown to follow an extension of total sleep time. Sleep insufficiency is sometimes confused with insomnia, but the opportunity to sleep differs in the two disorders (with insomnia sufferers typically being unable to sleep despite having opportunities to do so)."[211]

By now, everyone knows that good-quality sleep is critical for physical and mental well-being. In contrast, insufficient sleep causes a range of medical issues. In earlier chapters, we discussed the various hormones that we need to monitor for good health. All of them function in delicate balance and change based on diet, exercise, and sleep patterns.

Genetic influences are also a factor. These influences may be at play in as many as one-third of those who suffer from insufficient sleep.[212] We know that our biological clock is embedded in our DNA, which controls our natural circadian rhythm to wake up and fall asleep.

Definition: Insomnia

The ICSD-3 defines insomnia as "a predominant complaint of dissatisfaction with sleep quantity or quality, associated with one (or more) of the following symptoms:

1. Difficulty initiating sleep. (In children, this may manifest as difficulty initiating sleep without caregiver intervention.)

2. Difficulty maintaining sleep, characterized by frequent awakenings or problems returning to sleep after awakenings. (In children, this may manifest as difficulty returning to sleep without caregiver intervention.)
3. Early-morning awakening with inability to return to sleep.

"The criteria includes not only a primary complaint of difficulty initiating sleep, maintaining sleep, waking too early, or un-restorative or poor quality sleep, but also that the sleep difficulty occurs despite adequate opportunity and circumstances for sleep, and that one or more complaints of daytime impairment are due to the sleep difficulty.

"The insomnia disorders can be either primary or secondary. Primary insomnias can have both intrinsic and extrinsic factors involved in their etiology, but they are not regarded as being secondary to another disorder. Secondary forms occur when the insomnia is a symptom of a medical or psychiatric illness, another sleep disorder, or substance abuse."[213]

The Prevalence of Insomnia

The prevalence of insomnia in working people is usually 23.2%, but it is significantly higher in women (27%) compared to men (19%). Women often begin to experience insomnia in adolescence, and this group develops worsening insomnia after menopause.[214, 215]

The elderly, individuals with low socioeconomic status, and those with poor health or low quality-of-life scores also experience higher rates of insomnia.[216, 217]

Chronic Insomnia

As noted earlier, 40% to 70% of people with acute insomnia can transition to chronic insomnia. Factors that increase the risk for chronic insomnia include[218]:

*   **Predisposition to insomnia.** Generally, these factors – such as personality traits and genetics, including family history – are not easily modifiable.

- *Precipitating acute event*. Often, a stressful life event related to family, work, or school acts as a major contributor.
- *Perpetuating variables*. Ongoing behaviors and coping strategies, such as substance abuse (discussed later in this chapter), can increase insomnia.

Five Stages of Sleep

Although we think of sleep as a time to "shut down," the brain is far from resting when we slip into slumber. Our brain's cortex is still running. Sleeping is not a passive process but rather an active metabolic process that repairs damaged cells, restores energy levels, and categorizes information gathered during the day and stores it into retrievable memory.

According to the American Association of Sleep Medicine, there are five progressive stages of sleep, beginning with non-rapid-eye movement (non-REM) sleep and ending with rapid-eye-movement (REM) sleep.

- Stage W (wakefulness)
- Stage 1 (Non-REM relaxed wakefulness)
- Stage 2 (Non-REM light sleep)
- Stage 3 (Non-REM deep or slow-wave sleep)
- Stage 4 (REM sleep or dreaming)

Stages 1 to 3 are non-REM sleep phases: cortical activity is low. During Stage 4, or REM sleep, the brain is highly active.[219]

We move through one complete cycle of sleep every 90 minutes (approximately). Non-REM sleep comprises 75% of this cycle. Our body relaxes, and our temperature, heart rate, and blood pressure all drop, and our cells repair, recover, and regenerate. To achieve sleep that is restorative and supportive to overall health, you also need to experience approximately 13% to 23% of your sleep in Stage 3, or deep sleep.[220]

In contrast, during REM sleep, the brain is very active, and energy is renewed in the brain and throughout the body. New brain neuro-connections are made. In doing so, our brains imprint memory and enable further learning. Without good sleep, it's harder to retain information.

REM sleep increases as the night continues, especially in the last third. As the sleep cycle progresses, Stage 2 begins to account for most non-REM sleep, and Stages 3 and 4 may disappear altogether.

Sleep experts define a good night of sleep as one that cycles through at least four and ideally five cycles of non-REM and REM sleep (this explains the recommendation of 7 to 8 hours of sleep, or five cycles of 90 minutes, totaling 7.5 hours). You are far better off having at least four cycles of sleep during the night, totaling 6 hours, than 8 hours of interrupted sleep.[221] Ideally, you should wake up naturally, without the need for an alarm clock. We all know the feeling of being jolted out of sleep when the buzzer goes off.

Effects of Insufficient Sleep on Health

Many biomarker levels are altered due to insufficient sleep. For example, cholesterol metabolism is altered, pro-inflammatory markers IL-1 and 6 increase, leptin lowers, and ghrelin increases. (Leptin and ghrelin are two hormones that influence our energy balance by suppressing and increasing hunger, respectively.) These hormones help us control our food energy needs to keep us at a healthy weight.[222, 223, 224]

The consequences of insufficient sleep include increased incidences of cardiovascular deaths and disease (including hypertension), obesity leading to diabetes, cancer, impaired cognitive functions, mental health issues, motor vehicle accidents, and accidents at workplaces, to just name of few.[225]

Impact on Metabolism

In the short term, insomnia leads to a cascade of metabolic reactions, such as higher blood sugar levels and insulin secretion, which adds to an increased glycation potential. Fred Turek, director of the Center for Sleep and Circadian Biology at Northwestern University, concluded that "short sleepers" are those who slept less than 6 hours a night and were 89% more likely to become obese and 28% more likely to develop diabetes. Turek also outlined that the difference between having a sleep debt and being fully rested is equivalent to consuming 1,000 fewer calories over 3 days.[226]

Another study researching the metabolic consequences of sleep deprivation also identifies short sleep as a cause of obesity.[227]

Insufficient sleep also reduces non-REM sleep and REM sleep, which has been associated with insulin resistance and can lead to diabetes in the longer term.[228]

These studies demonstrate the link between sleep and metabolic health. Therefore, overweight and obese people who want to lose weight must eat less, exercise more, and sleep well.[229]

Impact on the Immune System

Sleep deprivation can negatively affect the immune system's ability to robustly mount a fight against infection. A study at the San Diego Veterans Affairs Medical Center showed that sleep-deprived men had substantially reduced white blood cell activity. These cells are necessary to protect the body from viruses and bacteria.[230]

Another study showed that those who do not sleep well experience respiratory infections more frequently.[231] This makes sense, considering the impact that sleep has on cortisol and how this hormone feeds our fight-or-flight response against both physical and mental stressors.

Impact on Cancer

As a society, we have seen a rise in cancer in the past decade, partly because we live longer than we used to and perhaps because we live in a more toxic environment, full of artificial chemicals. However, studies also show that insufficient sleep, including short sleep duration and sleep disruption, might increase a person's risk of cancer, especially of the prostate and breast.[232]

We know that sleep improves our immune system, and a lack of sleep compromises it. Many oncologists believe that the rise in cancer incidence is connected to our inability to rid our bodies of cancer cells. It has also been suggested that the hormone melatonin is involved in the relationship between sleep and cancer, especially breast cancer.[233] Read more about melatonin later in this chapter.

Impact on Mood

There is no doubt people feel "moody" when they haven't had enough sleep. The changes to the quality and quantity of our sleep during the pandemic have exacerbated how emotionally unwell we feel now.[234]

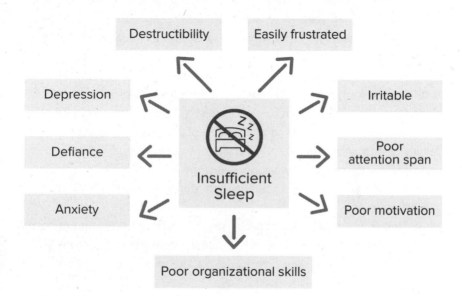

Insomnia strongly predicts depression, since 90% of patients with major depressive disorder (MDD) have difficulty sleeping. Sleep disturbances are part of the diagnostic criteria for depression and generalized anxiety disorder, but if insomnia is a coexisting disorder, it worsens prognosis.[235]

Some mental health experts believe that insomnia exacerbates depression and post-traumatic stress disorder (PTSD), which drives the suicide epidemic in veterans.[236, 237]

Effects of Insufficient Sleep on the Workplace

Mood changes and depression symptoms can certainly impact teamwork and productivity. We know that shift workers, especially those who have formal shift work, are at increased risk for sleep insufficiency. Studies have shown these workers are at high risk for cardiometabolic stress and cognitive impairment resulting in accidents.[238] How many times have we heard that a "human error" was to blame for a workplace accident?

This is a huge issue for the manufacturing and transportation industries.[239, 240] One study demonstrated that those workers who averaged about 5.6 hours of sleep were found to have impaired reaction time, to perform twice as slow (especially at night), and to have a fivefold lapse decrease in attention.[241]

We are also acutely aware that when we are sleepy, we don't "think" as well. Research supports this, showing that we have reduced active cognitive process capabilities, such as planning, coping, and problem-solving. This translates into deficits in analyzing unfamiliar environmental challenges or sustaining an extended chain of logical thought. All of us are trying to figure out new working solutions during this pandemic and for when it ends, and such impairments do not support creativity and productivity.

It's worth noting that sleep problems are an initial symptom of burnout.[242, 243] Therefore, all of us should make it a strong priority to find ways to monitor and support good sleep during the pandemic and beyond.

> "Every important mistake I've made in my life I made when I was tired."[244]
>
> — *Former U.S. president Bill Clinton*

Effects of Insufficient Sleep on Vulnerable Communities, Veterans, and Those with PTSD

A U.S. Department of Veterans Affairs study found that more than 90% of people who have experienced acute life trauma have sleep issues. Not only do they have insomnia, but they also endure nightmares.[245]

Alcohol and Substance Abusers

In Chapter 2, we discussed the increased use of alcohol and recreational drugs during this pandemic. People who used alcohol, cannabis, and pre-scription drugs to support their sleep routines before COVID-19 leaned into them more. However, the interactions between these types of drugs and insomnia are complex. Approximately 15% to 30% of people use alcohol to manage their insomnia. Unfortunately, people can develop a dependence on and tolerance to the sedative effects of alcohol, which can lead to a higher quantity consumed and even alcoholism.[246]

Alcohol can also impact the quality of sleep. Many of my clients who abstain from alcohol during a cleanse often comment that they experi-ence better sleep. Insomnia in alcohol-dependent people is estimated at 36% to 91%.

The use of cannabis has been beneficial for some people who might have imbalances in their neurotransmitter levels. In my practice, people who have low serotonin or low GABA can improve their sleep by taking supplements that boost these two neurotransmitters. However, those who use cannabis can also develop dependency and tolerance, just like with long-term alcohol use. Daily cannabis users have a higher rate of sleep disturbances and, when abstaining, can develop severe insomnia. Notable symptoms include trouble falling asleep and staying asleep, and vivid dreams – all of which make it difficult to quit.[247, 248]

Menopausal Women

Ask a group of perimenopausal women how well they sleep, and most will answer, "Not well at all, if at all." We know that insomnia strikes women more than men, and chronic insomnia symptoms do increase with the severity of hot flashes and night sweats. Eighty percent of women with severe vasomotor symptoms, such as hot flashes and night sweats, experience insomnia.[249]

The Aged

There is no doubt that biological factors related to aging impact the elderly and their ability to sleep. It is not uncommon that people feel frustrated by this, given that poor sleep leads to poor energy and brain fog. As we age, there is an interruption to our circadian rhythm, or our biological clock. Sleep experts have determined that elderly people experience less deep sleep, more sleep fragmentation, and early-morning awakening. And because melatonin secretion falls as we get older, it is common for older people to experience sleep disorders.

Precipitating factors include preexisting health problems (for example, nighttime urination, labored breathing, pain), lifestyle changes after retirement (and during lockdowns), poor physical function, concurrent medications, and – more recently – worsening social isolation.[250, 251, 252, 253]

How to Get Enough Quality Sleep

There are many ways to improve sleep. Let us explore some of the more recent ideas to reduce insomnia risk.[254]

Sleep Hygiene

There has been a lot of research done on the effects of bedtime screen use and our need to reduce the use of devices at least 1 to 2 hours before we sleep. The bright blue light from devices stimulates wakefulness because it interferes with the natural secretion of melatonin.[255] Children and adolescents are particularly sensitive to this light, with almost twice the melatonin suppression compared to adults.[256]

Today, many devices include a nighttime setting that changes the screen lighting to a different wavelength of color. Set it to change at least 2 hours before your natural bedtime.

Cognitive and Behavioral Therapy

The goal is simple: to break the unhealthy connection between the bed and thoughts of insomnia. Staying awake, being frustrated, and worried about trying to fall asleep can, in fact, cause a hyperarousal state. Try to limit the time you're awake in bed. Many therapists recommend getting out of bed if you can't sleep, and resetting by doing things like reading a book. Set realistic expectations about the amount and quality of sleep you can achieve based on your current environmental status, such as the stress you're feeling about your work and home life situations, your access to healthy food, and your ability to exercise regularly.

In addition to good sleep hygiene, consider cognitive and behavior therapy (CBT) if you are having sleep issues and can't achieve better sleep on your own. This kind of therapy is scientifically effective for the treatment of insomnia.[257]

Using sleep medications, such as benzodiazepines, can be helpful for short-term acute situations but can be addictive over time.[258] The good news is, CBT has far more sustained long-term results than drug therapy for "curing" insomnia.

Darkness

People tend to sleep more in extreme northern and southern climates during the winter months because they don't see as much sunlight. Many people suffer from sleep disorders that are related to a lack of sunlight. In contrast, during the summer months, we all seem to have more energy and feel less sleepy with longer and sunnier days.

Visually impaired people often suffer from sleep disorders too – they have lost their light-triggering mechanism to regulate their melatonin levels (read more about melatonin below). Nightshift workers are also prone to imbalanced melatonin levels, since they often sleep during the sunny stretches of the day.

It's essential to keep your sleep space dark and your devices out of the bedroom. And if you can't, try an eye shield.

Coolness

Ideally, your bedroom should also be cool when you sleep. Simply lowering the temperature in your bedroom and cooling the body by (0.3°C to

0.4°C) promotes drowsiness. A room temperature that hovers between 65°F and 70°F (19°C and 21°C) is ideal.[259]

To bring your body temperature down before bed, take a warm bath or shower. It sounds counterintuitive, but the warm water increases your core temperature initially (which helps melatonin production) and then your body's peripheral blood vessels widen to release body heat and bring your overall body temperature down. This vasodilation effect mimics the effect of melatonin.

Melatonin levels increase when warm bath water is heated by as little as 3.6°F (2°C). That's why having a warm bath or shower before bed is a great way to relax and get to sleep. Ninety minutes before bed, take a shower with the water temperature at 104°F to 109°F (40°C to 43°C), as this can help you fall asleep an average of 10 minutes more quickly.[260]

Other methods of cooling down include pressing cold facecloths to your wrists and the back of your neck, arranging a fan (or fans) in your bedroom to increase airflow, sucking on ice cubes, and choosing low-thread-count cotton sheets, which are more breathable – and therefore cooler – than other options.

Supplements as a Sleep Aid

MELATONIN

Much has already been said about the effects of melatonin on our wake–sleep cycle. But melatonin has many other vital functions, notably as an antioxidant and detoxifier of free radicals and for its impact on the prevention and treatment of cancer. Other positive physiological effects include bone formation and protection; reproductive, cardiovascular and immune health; and body mass regulation. Many scientists have also studied its potential protective effects on the brain and gastrointestinal system and its use in the treatment of some psychiatric disorders.[261]

Melatonin stimulates the release of several other hormones in the body, including growth hormone and sex hormones. It is during REM sleep that growth hormone is released. The secretion of melatonin slowly declines as we age, and when we reach around age 45, it dramatically drops, causing an increase in sleep issues.

Melatonin is produced in the gut during the day (hence the importance of good gut health) and in our brain's pineal gland at night. The
hormone is made from tryptophan. We get tryptophan from the foods
we eat. Tryptophan is found in meat and poultry, but the richest sources
are sunflower seeds, pumpkin seeds, collard greens, turnip greens, and
especially potatoes (with the skins) and bananas. Once tryptophan is
consumed, the body converts it into the neurotransmitter serotonin. At
night, serotonin is converted into melatonin.

Melatonin can be purchased as a supplement. It appears to be safe
to use in low doses. Its side effects include drowsiness, lower body temperature, and vivid dreams; some people may also experience blood
pressure changes (blood pressure can lower if you're healthy, and it may
increase with certain medications).

It would be best if you took melatonin under the supervision of a
health professional familiar with dosing and the different sources of
melatonin; melatonin is not a regulated substance, and almost anyone
can manufacture it. But some formulations may be of poor quality or
impure, increasing your risk of side effects.

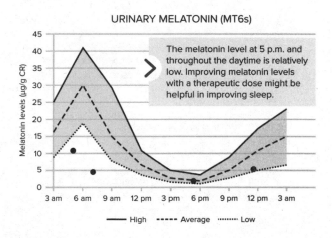

URINARY MELATONIN (MT6s)

> The melatonin level at 5 p.m. and throughout the daytime is relatively low. Improving melatonin levels with a therapeutic dose might be helpful in improving sleep.

——— High   – – – – Average   ········ Low

GABA

Neurotransmitters, as we discussed in Chapter 5, are critical to regulating
sleep. Gamma-aminobutyric acid (GABA) is the neurotransmitter that
promotes sleep. Norepinephrine (triggered by cortisol) and dopamine

promote wakefulness. Serotonin is necessary for both optimal sleep and wakefulness.

This model of the sleep–wake cycle is often called the flip-flop switch because it permits a person to be either awake or asleep, but not both at the same time.[262]

GABA is synthesized from glutamate, another neurotransmitter, and vitamin B_6 (found in fortified cereals, beef, poultry, and starchy vegetables).

People with low levels of GABA may experience difficulty sleeping. And stress can compound the problem because our body may redirect our glutamine (required to make GABA) to manufacture instead more glutathione, an important antioxidant that reduces oxidative damage due to stress.

GABA dosing can start at 200 mg and be gradually increased under the guidance of a healthcare professional. Additional glutamine or glutathione may be added for those who are deficient.

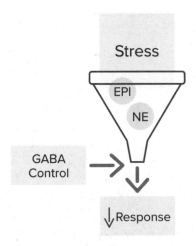

Herbs as Nervines

For thousands of years, before manufactured drugs were developed, many cultures used botanicals to treat illness. Nervines (nerve tonics) from the botanical world can help with insomnia.

While some of the herbs help support relaxation, others can act as sedatives or hypnotics, which promote deep sleep. Nervines can also support weakened or overworked adrenal glands (which excrete cortisol) at times of acute stress and during fatigue caused by longer-term stress conditions.

CHAMOMILE

Matricaria chamomilla has a long history in many cultures and has been used in tea format to reduce anxiety, support sleep, and settle gastrointestinal discomforts. Its sedative effects are likely induced by its regulating effect on the GABA receptor. Also, small concentrations of GABA can be found in this plant.[263]

Chamomile was also shown to reduce generalized anxiety when used in the long term; one study claimed the efficacy of chamomile was comparable to conventional anxiolytic (antianxiety) drugs without the adverse side effects.[264]

The standard starting dose is about 400 mg oral capsules of chamomile twice daily.[265]

Chamomile appears to be safe in higher doses. Postpartum mothers took up to 2000 mg to support sleep without adverse side effects.[266]

VALERIANS

Valeriana officinalis is a well-understood herb that is used as an effective mild sedative. Trials show that valerian helped participants fall asleep, improving their sleep continuity, and decreased restlessness and tension.[267]

The likely mechanism for these effects is not the small amount of GABA found in valerian but rather its effect on modulating GABA receptors.

Using valerian and Saint-John's-wort (another herb) under a naturopathic doctor's supervision can be an effective alternative to a sedative prescription drug class of benzodiazepines.[268] Effects are not immediate; symptoms improve after ingesting the herb for 2 weeks.

The starting dose of valerian when used on its own is 400 to 900 mg.

HOPS

Humulus lupulus is part of the hemp family, which we know is related to cannabis. It is used to make beer but is also used to support sleep. Hops work most effectively as a sleep aid when used in conjunction with valerian.[269] However, hops should be used cautiously in people with depression, given it is part of the cannabis plant family and can negatively impact those with clinical depression.

The suggested starting dose of valerian combined with hops is 187 to 250 mg valerian plus 42 to 60 mg hops.

KAVA

Piper methysticum was discovered in the Pacific Islands, and natives consume this kava root by chewing it or mixing it in grounded form with a fluid; it's used during religious ceremonies to help worshippers reach higher states of consciousness.

Kava has been shown to decrease anxiety and promote relaxation without a loss of mental acuity. Studies suggest that kava acts on GABA receptors to reduce light sleep and lengthen deep sleep.[270]

An effective dose of kava ranges from 70 to 250 mg per day.

PASSIONFLOWER

Passiflora incarnata is found in many supplement formulas because of its proven effects in reducing tension and nerve pain and treating insomnia. Holistic practitioners like it because it does not have a hangover effect.

Clinical studies confirm its positive impact on quality of sleep and anxiety reduction. It appears that the pathway for these effects is its modulation on the GABA receptors.[271, 272, 273]

The starting dose of ingesting passionflower as a tea or in dried capsule form is 0.25 to 2.00 g up to three times a day.

LAVENDER

Lavendula officinalis is not only a beautiful plant, but it's also loved by many as a classic aroma in spas. But this sweet-scented plant has medicinal qualities too. It is used to relieve stress and exhaustion and to treat sleep disorders, headaches, parasitic infections, burns, insect bites, and spasms.[274]

In studies, a 6-week use of an oral lavender oil preparation (silexan, 80 mg/day) showed it effectively reduced generalized anxiety comparable to a 0.5 mg per-day dose of lorazepam (a prescription benzodiazepine often called Ativan).[275] Similarly, a 2% concentration of lavender oil used as aromatherapy was found to help support the treatment of anxiety and depression.[276]

Lavender's calming action appears to be from its impact on both the GABA and dopaminergic receptors.

Most herbalists would suggest ingesting lavender, but many use it in aromatherapy. There is no evidence of toxicity with short-term use; therefore, use it freely!

Power Napping

We accept the importance of sleep for top performers, such as athletes, musicians, and pilots, many of whom nap before their big day or important task. Many take naps regularly and get more than half an hour more sleep daily.

The space agency NASA found that pilots who power-napped had up to 54% improved alertness compared to pilots who didn't nap. The recommendation is not to over-nap. Limit naps to 10 to 20 minutes.[277]

If you have difficulty napping, not to worry. Just close your eyes and meditate for the same amount of time to let your mind rest.

Summary: How to Get Enough Quality Sleep

1. Go to sleep at the same time each day to establish a regular circadian (sleep–wake) rhythm.
2. Expose yourself to adequate amounts of sunlight during the day.
3. Avoid stimulants (caffeine, energy drinks, amphetamines), including vigorous exercise after 5 p.m.
4. Don't nap late in the day – power naps of 10 to 20 minutes midday work best.
5. Avoid large and heavy meals after 8 p.m., and stop snacking after dinner.

6. Avoid alcohol before sleeping – it may knock you out, but it will also keep you from leaving REM light-sleep stage.
7. Relax before bed by playing soft music, reading a fiction book, or meditating.
8. Shut down the electronic devices and TVs at least 1 hour before bedtime. Keep them out of the bedroom altogether.
9. Create an environment conducive for sleeping – a quiet, dark, and cooler-temperature room.
10. Have a warm bath or shower 90 minutes before bed to stimulate melatonin for sleep.

If these tips don't help and you can't sleep properly, try a supplement recommended by your healthcare professional or consult your doctor, who may prescribe a sleep medication. Note that most prescription drugs can be habit-forming, and nearly all are associated with some form of side effect. Long-term use is not recommended.

Myths and Facts about Sleep

Myth 1: Getting just an hour less sleep a night won't affect your daytime functioning. You may not feel sleepy during the day, but losing just 1 hour of shut-eye will impact your ability to think and respond effectively. Remember the importance of completing at least four cycles of sleep.

Myth 2: Your body can adjust to different sleep schedules. The truth is, most people can reset their biological clock by only 1 to 2 hours a day. This is why it can take more than a week to adjust your biological clock after traveling across several time zones or switching back and forth from a day shift to a night shift.

Myth 3: Catch-up sleep can cure excessive daytime fatigue. This may be true to some degree, but it's not just the quantity of sleep, it's also the *quality* of sleep that you must pay attention to. To get more mind- and mood-boosting REM sleep, try sleeping an extra 30 minutes to 1 hour in the morning, when REM sleep stages are longer. Improving your overall sleep will also increase your REM sleep. If you aren't getting enough deep sleep, your body will try to make that up first, at the expense of REM sleep.

Myth 4: You can make up lost sleep hours during the week by being a weekend sleeper. Although this will help relieve some sleep debt, it will not ultimately make up for the lack of sleep. Sleeping longer on weekends can affect your sleep–wake cycle, making it harder to go to sleep at the right time on Sunday nights and to get up early on Monday mornings.

CHAPTER 10

Beyond Being Active

Everyone knows the importance of staying active and working out. There are so many reasons to exercise. Not only does it keep your heart healthy, it also contributes to the health of your lungs, muscles, bones, immune system, brain, and, therefore, your mental well-being. Because of lockdowns, we have been forced out of our regular activities – whether it's going window-shopping with friends, participating in gym and yoga classes, or vacationing on cycling trips. Unfortunately, finding even simple skipping ropes, free weights, and bicycles has been difficult, with supplies out of stock for much of the pandemic.

It's well documented in the scientific literature that regular exercise can reduce the onset of age-related cardiovascular disease, hypertension, and diabetes. But until recently, there was very little molecular evidence to link exercise with a reduction in your overall risk for disease and your chances of living a longer life. Telomere length may provide that missing thread of molecular evidence (more about telomeres in the next chapter).

The bonus is, the more you move, the more calories you burn, which means you can enjoy some treats from time to time. But exercising does not zero out a high-calorie, bad-quality diet; you can't just burn off all the extra calories you might eat. Some people say, "I exercise to eat and drink." Do not fall into this trap! What's more important is making healthy food choices and eating in moderation.

And for those who think they can replace sleep with exercise to feel more energetic, you are wrong. As you read in the previous chapter, you can't cheat sleep. It would be best if you put in the hours to give your body the rest it needs to repair, recover, and renew.

It's important to understand that fitness and exercise are not necessarily the same thing. Many people exercise, but they're not fit and healthy. Their exercise is inadequate and doesn't stimulate the metabolic changes they need to maintain or improve their health.

Being fit and embracing a healthy lifestyle has so many positive effects on the body. For example, studies have shown that exercising:

- Decreases cardiovascular inflammation by lowering blood pressure and cholesterol levels
- Reduces the risk of diabetes by lowering excessive blood glucose and insulin, which prevents glycation
- Increases antiaging hormones, such as growth hormone, testosterone, and serotonin
- Induces the body's antioxidants, which reduces oxidative stress

Exercise routines have changed for a lot of people during the pandemic. Those who regularly went to the gym had to stop. Even the Olympians had to find innovative ways to train. The good news is, some people chose to keep exercising or found ways to start exercising, making good use of any extra time they had on hand.

We have seen mental health issues skyrocket to new levels since the onset of the pandemic. And studies have shown again and again that physical activity and exercise remain some of the most effective strategies for treating the symptoms of anxiety and depression.

However, here is a stark reality: the pandemic impacted our essential baseline, our step count. Ten days after the pandemic was declared by the World Health Organization on March 11, 2020, there was a 5.5% decrease in mean daily step count (287 steps) worldwide, which grew to a 27.0% reduction (1,432 steps) within 30 days. Indeed, geographical areas that were not as impacted with lockdowns showed better daily step counts.[278]

Many of us had to transition to working from home, which cut back on our steps to and from work and around the office. We had to have all our meetings over Zoom and Microsoft Teams. New discomforts and strains took hold. Our backs and hips began to hurt as we sat for hours. And as we typed endlessly on our keyboards, our neck and shoulders stiffened, and our wrists and thumbs became sore.

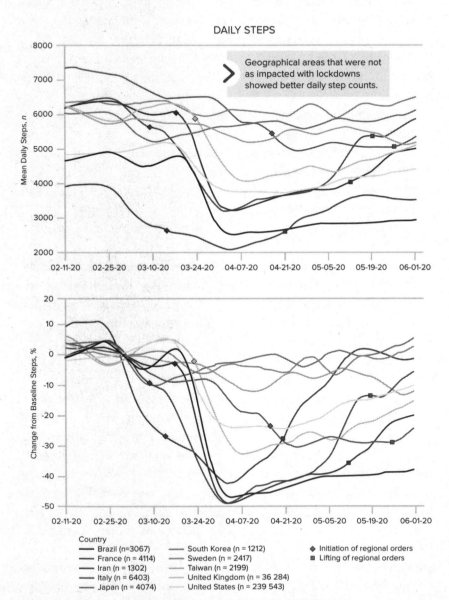

DAILY STEPS

Geographical areas that were not as impacted with lockdowns showed better daily step counts.

Country
— Brazil (n=3067)   — South Korea (n = 1212)   ◆ Initiation of regional orders
— France (n = 4114)   — Sweden (n = 2417)   ■ Lifting of regional orders
— Iran (n = 1302)   ⋯ Taiwan (n = 2199)
— Italy (n = 6403)   United Kingdom (n = 36 284)
— Japan (n = 4074)   United States (n = 239 543)

Source: Ann Intern Med. 2020; 173(9):767-770. doi:10.7326/M20-2665

Working from Home

Earlier in the book, I spoke about the extra work hours that were added to a workday at home. A Harvard Business School study analyzed anonymous emails and meeting invitations of 3.1 million employees at 21,500 companies in North America, Europe, and the Middle East. Here were their findings[279]:

- The average workday increased by 8.2%, or 48.5 minutes.
- People wrote 5.2% more emails a day, and 8.3% were sent after business hours.
- Team members attended 13% more meetings.
- The number of people invited to each meeting rose by 14%, or two extra people.

Not surprisingly, both Zoom and Microsoft Teams users increased exponentially. Note: The April statistics include students' online learning.

Zoom & Microsoft Teams Users

Month	Daily Zoom Users	Daily Teams Users
December 2019	10 million	20 million
March 2020	200 million	44 million
April 2020	300 million	75 million

The Different Kinds of Exercise

There are three core areas of physical activity:

1. Aerobic, or cardio exercise
2. Anaerobic, or strength training
3. NEAT movement, or non-exercise activity thermogenesis

The two main types of exercise – aerobic and anaerobic – affect the essential aging-related hormones in all of us. One type of exercise doesn't replace the other.

Aerobic exercise includes activities such as jogging, walking, and going up and down stairs. These types of actions improve your cardiac fitness and pulmonary function – they're crucial for maintaining your quality of life.

Anaerobic exercise usually involves resistance. Weightlifting and Pilates are the most popular types of resistive training. This type of exercise improves your lean body mass, prevents bone loss, strengthens your tendons and ligaments, and increases your basic metabolic rate.

NEAT movements are the activities of your daily living – slipping in and out of your chair, standing up to do some work or light chores around the house, and unfocused amounts of miscellaneous walking (below we discuss yoga and tai chi as NEAT movements as well).

A general physical activity guideline suggests that an average adult should aim for:

- At least 150 to 300 minutes per week of moderate aerobic physical activity or 75 minutes of vigorous-intensity per week
- Two sessions of muscle strength training per week
- A NEAT activity every day

How Can You Exercise at Home?

- Use any exercise equipment you have, such as weights, a treadmill, elliptical machine, and stationary bike.
- Non-equipment aerobic exercise ideas include speed walking, jogging, jumping jacks, hiking, skipping rope, dancing, going up and down stairs in your home or apartment building, and going for a bike ride.
- Housework counts for physical activity as well, such as landscaping, vacuuming, and cleaning floors.
- Try standing squats, push-ups, and sit-ups to build muscle strength.
- Carry textbooks, canned goods, jugs filled with water, and paint cans around as a form of weight training.
- Stretch while you are watching TV or a movie.

Need motivation? Download a fitness app or an online platform to get a trainer into your private space on your own time and to keep you focused and on track. This works especially well when you lack the motivation or know-how to do it on your own. Better still, enroll with a family member or friend to develop a routine and enforce some accountability to each other.

Overall, that is about 30 minutes of movement five times per week. It is also okay to break it up into five-, 10-, 15-, or 20-minute allotments. Schedule it in your calendar!

I've taken up an idea I learned from Dr. Sanjay Gupta, CNN's chief medical correspondent. When I interviewed him about his book for *Macleans* magazine years ago, I asked him how he was able to fit working out into his schedule. His solution? He schedules his vigorous aerobic workouts into his calendar, and they don't get moved. He also does a lot of his strength training and walking while doing his calls.

TIP: If you do not need to do your meetings over Zoom or Teams, then just use the phone. This way, you can get out of your chair to walk, do stretches, or lift some light weights. It's not ideal, but it's better than nothing, especially if you don't have time to fit it all in.

Aerobic Exercise, or Cardio

There are all kinds of ways to get your aerobic exercise. Depending on the state of your home, some would say that vacuuming and cleaning your floors counts as cardio! What works well and can save you time is a group of aerobic activities know as high-intensity interval training, or HIIT. I am a huge fan of HIIT. Many new workout trends are based on this model because they are quick and effective, raise your metabolic rate, and burn fat. The additional benefit is what many trainers call afterburn, which means calories continue to burn even after you stop exercising. It works by shifting your body back and forth between aerobic mode, which uses a lot of oxygen, and anaerobic mode, where you use stored energy.[280]

To do a HIIT workout, alternate steady movement with faster movement. A typical HIIT training session would involve short bursts (from 6 seconds to 4 minutes) of intense exercise (greater than or equal to 90% maximal aerobic capacity, which essentially means you are very short of breath and at 90% of your ideal maximum heart rate based on age) alternated with relief breaks of various lengths, to slow down your heart rate and breathing. People can lose almost 30% more weight doing HIIT than with more traditional aerobic exercising. Aim for 20 to 30 minutes of this type of workout at least three times a week.[281]

Maximum Heart Rates While Exercising

To see an improvement in your cardiovascular and pulmonary functions, make sure you perform your activity at 55% to 65% of your maximum heart rate. Track your heart rate with a wearable device. You can calculate maximum heart rates by subtracting your chronological age from 220 for a man, and from 216 for a woman.

Use the following formulas to calculate your maximum heart rate:

Male: 220 − (0.55 x age)
Female: 216 − (1.09 x age)

For example: a 40-year-old woman's rate would be 172.4, or 216 − (1.09 x 40).

Adults can improve their cardiorespiratory fitness (VO2max) from 4% to 46% in training periods lasting from 2 to 15 weeks with HIIT. Insulin sensitivity can also be improved by 23% to 58% in that same time frame.[282]

HDL ("good") cholesterol rises within 8 weeks of training.[283] You can see the many benefits of HIIT and why I love to use this form of exercise in my personal routine.

Here are some positive metabolic effects of HIIT[284]:

- The heart rate elevates significantly, exercising your heart muscle.
- The sympathetic nervous system (which speeds up neural signaling

messages) is elevated. Epinephrine and norepinephrine elevate 6.2 to 14.5 times greater than baseline, which boosts your energy after exercising.

- Initially, blood glucose (from glycogen breakdown) is elevated (for exercise fuel), but it may decline during a HIIT session.
- Increased ATP (adenosine triphosphate) translates into an increase of mitochondrial biogenesis; this is the energy used to meet the rapid fuel needs of your contracting muscles, such as those of the heart.
- Blood glycerol and free fatty acid levels increase, suggesting an early breakdown of triglycerides, which lowers the risk of insulin resistance.
- Growth hormone may increase up to 10 times above baseline, acting as a repair hormone.
- Venous blood return to the heart is enhanced, directly increasing stroke volume and reducing diastolic blood pressure.

Note: Those who have a cardiac condition must consult with their doctor before starting HIIT, as some of these effects can negatively impact a weak heart.

Anaerobic Exercise, or Strength Training

Trainers recommend starting with aerobic exercise followed by anaerobic exercise. This is because the pituitary gland in your brain releases a surge of human growth hormone within 30 minutes of a run or equivalent activity, peaking for approximately 15 to 20 minutes. This burst helps to repair damaged muscles and increases your muscle mass. It also helps to burn body fat. Your insulin levels also drop, and glucagon – another hormone – rises. Both hormones stimulate another release of growth hormone. More testosterone and growth hormone are released into your bloodstream within 5 minutes of weightlifting, and these can linger for another 30 minutes. As you'll recall, these hormones are essential for repairing muscles, bones, and tissues and they boost the immune system so that it functions at its peak ability.[285]

Building your muscles not only makes you look good with incredible body sculpting, but it also boosts your metabolism and gives your bones more support, like tree bark along a tree trunk. Muscle burns four times as many calories as fat, even at rest. The more muscle you have, the more you will burn. Men generally have more muscle than women, and therefore they have a faster metabolism and need to eat more and don't gain as much weight.[286]

Having more lean body mass or muscles reduces the incidence of insulin resistance and, therefore, metabolic syndrome.[287, 288] You'll recall that this increases the risk of cardiovascular disease and type 2 diabetes.

In addition to the many metabolic benefits, strength training also:

- Improves balance
- Enhances posture
- Increases coordination
- Prevents injury
- Protects bone health
- Slows age-related muscle loss

Trainers would recommend sessions that last between 45 and 60 minutes. And each movement type should be repeated eight to 10 times in one cycle. Perform each cycle three times. We often think of weight training when we think of anaerobic exercise, something we do in the gym. But remember that power yoga and bodyweight exercises are also excellent and they don't require equipment or membership fees!

Moderation Applies to Exercise Too

Is it possible to exercise too much? Should you be concerned about overtraining? Yes. I see this often in my practice.

What drives people to train for marathon after marathon or ride 100 miles a day for weeks? Multiple factors, I assure you. It often begins innocently, as a means of exercise or as a personal goal. Some people use it as a means of emotional escape or to fill up "empty" or "lonely" time. Before they know it, the endorphins kick in. These natural painkillers that the body secretes to decrease muscle pain also create a euphoric high, which becomes addictive. One of my patients told me that most people in his bike-riding group are exercise bulimics – purging calories through exercise. Riding long distances allows them to eat far too much and drink alcohol while staying slim. Although this highlights the psychology of overtraining, there are also many physical downsides of overtraining.

For example, heavy training may actually work against endurance athletes' health, resulting in skeletal muscle damage, as seen in one study conducted in South Africa.[289]

What exactly is overtraining? Let's just say that more than 60 minutes of aerobic and anaerobic exercise can create undesirable health side effects related to aging. Burning more than 2,000 calories a day doesn't help you live longer, even though it maintains your strength and functionality. Essentially, overtraining stresses your body, which causes the secretion of cortisol. This hormone shuts down many of the body's other hormones so that it can switch from growth-and-repair mode to fight-or-flight mode. Blood sugar rises (which is terrible for antiaging), and testosterone production drops in favor of cortisol production. This process creates less muscle mass and increases the risk of the cortisol-insulin cycle, impairing healthy metabolism.

We also know that exercise produces inflammatory proteins and free radicals. The body can handle the production of some of these – but too much can cause damage.[290]

Exercise and Nutrients

You can take certain nutrients and supplements before an exercise routine to boost growth hormone release and adenosine triphosphate (ATP) production.[291] For many years, I've recommended taking arginine, ornithine, and glutamine – all amino acids (derived from proteins) – to stimulate growth hormone in my patients with low levels of these amino acids. Ideally, you should take these amino acids 30 minutes before beginning exercise. A protein shake or bar might be an excellent option.

Athletes have used creatine supplements for many years because they act as an energy resource for skeletal muscles through the production of ATP. Some scientific studies report that creatine boosts your exercise response and endurance by 5% to 15%.[292, 293]

NEAT Movement

You should also consider non-exercise activity thermogenesis (NEAT) movement as part of your activity regimen, including stretching exercises. Dancing, tai chi, and yoga are all great examples. They can be performed daily for at least 30 minutes (start with 10 to 15 minutes each day). At the very least, this kind of movement improves your flexibility, which is critical to preventing injury as you get older, and it helps promote good spinal alignment and disk health. Movement and stretching exercises also have a rejuvenating effect, balancing sympathetic and parasympathetic tone in your nervous system, also known as the autonomic nervous system.

This system controls most of the unconscious functions in your body, such as your heart rate, breathing, swallowing, and sexual arousal. These are otherwise known as our primitive functions, and they are essential to our survival. Keeping the autonomic nervous system in good shape and in balance is necessary for life.

Yoga

Yoga, derived from the Sanskrit word *Yuji*, which means union, originated in India more than 5,000 years ago. It is an ancient practice that brings together mind and body. Many people consider it to be a spiritual tool that enhances health and well-being. It is comprised of postures (asanas), breathing (pranayama), and meditation.

Many people have embraced yoga since the pandemic hit, especially during the lockdowns. It's an activity you can do right at home. Beyond the benefits already outlined for NEAT movement in general, yoga helps us to stretch and it makes time to breathe and relax. I've finally been able to find the time to do yoga regularly and am proud to say I can touch my toes now!

Once upon a time, yoga was something "hippies" did, at least for my age group when I was in high school. Then yoga began to take hold as a healthy way to manage a busy life. Lululemon was established in Vancouver, Canada, in 1998, selling niche higher-quality yoga garments. Fast-forward to 2021, yoga has become what you "should do" to be on trend with folks who eat organic, drive green cars, and do not drink out of plastic bottles.

Lululemon

Lululemon is a global garment company that started as a niche yoga clothing company. Annual sales have been climbing as people stayed home during the pandemic. The company recorded a net income of about $329 million for the period ending January 31, 2021, up from $298 million in 2019.

A research team reviewed 81 studies to compare the effects of yoga and exercise. They found that yoga may be as effective or even more effective than exercise at improving a variety of health-related outcome measures.[294] *Wow*.

• Decreases stress and anxiety

One of the most popular reasons people start yoga is because they want to find a way to relax. Three months of yoga can lower levels of stress, anxiety, fatigue, and even depression.[295, 296] Technically, yoga does indeed decrease cortisol, especially when practiced alongside meditation.

• Reduces inflammation

As we discussed earlier, yoga can also protect against some chronic diseases, such as heart disease, cancer, and diabetes. Practitioners of yoga develop fewer inflammatory markers triggered by stress compared to non-practitioners.[297]

• Reduces cardiovascular disease risk

In one study, people who practiced yoga for at least 5 years had lower blood pressure compared to those who did not.[298]

In another study, as part of their cardiac rehabilitation program, patients who practiced yoga were able to lower their LDL ("bad") cholesterol and stop the progression of their disease.[299]

Certainly, additional lifestyle choices are likely associated with reducing these risk factors, but this is an excellent start. We often say that people who practice one healthy lifestyle choice will likely do more.

• Reduces chronic pain

Many people who have chronic musculoskeletal pain from arthritis in joints and in the back often use painkillers as their first choice of relief. But people who choose to practice yoga have been able to reduce their pain as well. It makes sense; the less flexible you become, the more frozen your joints become. Indeed, as noted above, pain increases cortisol, but a reduction of cortisol can reduce inflammatory markers.[300]

• Provides proprioception training

As we get older, we begin to experience reduced perception or awareness of the position and movement of our body; this is partly due to a loss of flexibility and muscle strength. We can all become more flexible, have better balance, and be stronger, though. These are critical factors needed to reduce falls and injury as we age. There is no doubt that sitting does not help our overall flexibility. Specific yoga poses challenge all these critical skills and improve our muscle strength, ligament elasticity, and bone density.[301, 302, 303]

• Supports weight loss

For many people, yoga may be the first activity they choose on their journey to become more active. Yoga does burn calories, especially hot yoga.[304] In fact, it can be quite a cardiac "workout." According to caloriesburnedhq.com, a person weighing 140 pounds (63.5 kg) who performs hatha yoga for 60 minutes would burn only around 177 calories, but someone weighing 200 pounds (91.7 kg) would burn 252 calories. If they both did hot yoga for the same amount of time, they would burn around 447 calories and 638 calories, respectively.

• Improves sleep

We have learned that nervines (from the botanical world) can support better sleep. One study put yoga practice against the use of Ayurvedic herbs. The research found that the yoga group fell asleep faster and stayed asleep longer than those who just used herbs.[305] This discovery may be helpful in geriatric groups where prescription drugs are overused to support sleep.

The mechanism of action is, you guessed it, the increased secretion of melatonin.[306]

In this 3-month study, the subjects in Group 1 served as controls. They did traditional flexibility exercises for 40 minutes and slow running for 20 minutes during the morning hours, and they played games for 60 minutes in the evening. Subjects in Group 2 practiced yoga: asanas (postures) for 45 minutes and pranayama (breathing exercises) for 15 minutes in the morning, and they also did yoga postures for 15 minutes, pranayama for 15 minutes, and meditation for 30 minutes before bed.

Beyond the increased melatonin secretion in Group 2, this group was also found to have a healthier heart rate, blood pressure, respiratory rate, and dynamic lung function. This study sums up the benefits of yoga.

Breathing

As we discussed, effectively exchanging gases in and out of our body is an important way to detoxify. Unfortunately, our lung capacity and lung function decrease after our mid-20s.

Breathing is not considered an exercise; we don't even think about doing it. It just happens, thanks to the autonomic functions controlled by our brain. Breathing requires many sets of muscles.

With chronic stress, these sets of muscles can get tight. You can't simply go to a massage therapist to do the stretching for you. Therefore, we need to breathe deeply to stretch them out and achieve maximum lung capacity. If you can control your breath, you are essentially in better control of your body.

Conscious breathing requires slow and methodical deep inhalations. Over time, this type of exercise improves pulmonary function and the delivery of oxygen to body tissues. It can also help improve cell waste removal – thereby controlling the body's acidity (pH levels) to allow cells to function better. Many benefits can be derived from breathing as part of meditation.

One study taught yoga poses, breathing techniques, and relaxation to college students in 50-minute classes twice a week. After 15 weeks, their lung vital capacity improved as measured using spirometry.[307]

Diaphragmatic Breathing

Like many others, I find it difficult to meditate without focusing on something. Try focusing on breathing.

How to do diaphragmatic, or "belly," breathing:

1. Sit back or lie down in a comfortable position.
2. Place one hand on your belly and the other hand on your chest.
3. Inhale through your nose and feel the air you are pushing into your belly. Feel your stomach expand.
4. Breathe out slowly through pursed lips and notice your belly go down. Breathe out twice as slowly as you breathe in.
5. Repeat.
6. Try this for 10 to 15 minutes per day.

By slowing down your breathing, you will keep your airways open longer, allowing your lungs to improve their exchange of oxygen and carbon dioxide by increasing the elasticity of the airways. In other words, you are actively stretching your lung tissues.

Tai Chi

Tai chi means "the ultimate of ultimate," which is often used to describe the vastness of the universe. This NEAT exercise, like yoga, can be done easily inside your home, in your backyard, or at the park.

When I was a child, I would be in awe as I watched seniors at the park rhythmically moving in unison from one pose to another. It was musical, and their flow was so calming. At that time, I wondered why these people chose to do this type of "exercise" with no cardio involved. I assumed it helped with their old-age stiffness. Fast-forward to my 50s, and welcome to my world of aging stiffness! Certainly, sitting for so many hours is not helpful.

Today, tai chi is one of the better-known flow practices. It was founded in China around 1670 and is based on both martial arts (shadowboxing) and qigong techniques. Philosophically, it is in line with Taoism, which focuses on the balance of opposites – physical and spiritual, yin and yang energies – and is characterized by contrast – slow versus fast, and soft versus hard.

Qigong and Tai Chi

Qigong is an ancient Chinese healing practice that promotes the movement of qi by opening gates and channels of energy in the body. It involves meditation, controlled breathing, and movement exercises.

Tai chi usually includes qigong concepts, but qigong practice would not necessarily include tai chi movements.

There are five different styles of tai chi; some are easier to master than others, but constant flow is common to all:

- Yang – relaxed, slow, and suitable for beginners
- Wu – very slow and focused on micro-movements
- Chen – uses both slow and fast movements, more advanced
- Sun - less kicking and punching than Chen, but similar
- Hao – not popular, focused on accurate positioning

Like acupuncture, tai chi has withstood the test of time. Recent scientific studies, predominantly with elderly subjects, demonstrate that tai chi has many health benefits.

- Improves cognitive function

Seniors often worry about losing their memory and their ability to perform executive functions as they grow old.

A study involving 60 older adults who did 50-minute tai chi sessions three times a week for 6 months showed measurable improvement in cognitive performance. The brain-derived neurotrophic factor (BDNF) inflammatory marker also decreased, which may be the mechanism to the improved brain function, since we know that inflammation in the brain plays a role in the deterioration of function.[308] We should seriously consider integrating tai chi into our lives!

• Decreases the risk of falls

When we are young, we take for granted that we have good balance. As we get older, we become weaker and less sturdy and are more likely to fall down, resulting in orthopedic and head trauma. These sorts of injuries can lead to increased bed rest, subsequent cardiovascular complications, and even death. Tai chi improves strength and balance with slow movements and constant poses.[309] It has been shown to be helpful in improving balance with patients who have Parkinson's disease.[310]

• Decreases stress and anxiety

Tai chi involves three modalities: exercise, breathing, and meditation. No wonder some researchers found that tai chi offered the same benefits as exercise in managing stress-related anxiety.[311]

• Improves sleep

It should be no surprise that people who practice this form of NEAT experience better-quality sleep. For those who suffer from anxiety, tai chi should be used as the first line of treatment before prescribing sleeping pills. Tai chi is also preferred over sleeping pill prescriptions for the elderly in retirement and nursing homes,[312] where group activities like tai chi can be organized.

• Reduces chronic pain

There is little doubt that movement "oils" the joints to prevent stiffness, which is the cornerstone to pain development. Regular practitioners of tai chi experience not only better mobility but also less pain.

Studies support this finding among osteoarthritic patients.[313] One of these studies found that tai chi was as effective as physiotherapy for knee pain.[314]

This concludes the section on approaches that can help you recover your body and mind. Since the onset of the pandemic, everything has seemed beyond our control. However, we can and must be disciplined with our lifestyle choices to support our recovery from the effects of COVID-19, even if we did not get infected. We all have become indirectly sick. Our overall physical health and mental well-being have suffered. If there is one thing we have learned, it's that our lifestyle choices impact how resilient we are against physical and mental challenges. In the final section of this book, I provide you with a compelling argument to take control of your health now, as it will impact not only your lifespan but also your health span.

RENEWING TO AN IMPROVED SELF

CHAPTER 11

Path to a Longer, Healthier Life

This chapter contains excerpts from my first book, *Lifeline: Unlock the Secrets of Your Telomeres for a Longer, Healthier Life.*

Twenty years ago, preventive medicine represented only a tiny part of the healthcare system, and personalized medicine was pretty much a dream. Today, both are respected and growing in influence, especially in the realms of cardiovascular, diabetes, and cancer treatment.

Within workplaces, organizations are just beginning to embrace a medical focus on their employees' physical health, safety, and mental well-being. COVID-19 has forced many leaders to acknowledge these essential variables to ensure a productive workplace. They are now using words like *prevention* and *resiliency* to describe how they are trying to take care of their employees and, at the same time, reduce healthcare benefits in an effort to reduce overall operating costs. However, developing resiliency requires investment in prevention health strategies.

But the bottom line remains the same for each of us. Everyone wants to know: How do we not get sick *and* never age?

Not everyone is a believer in medical prevention strategies. Some people ask me: "What evidence do you have that preventive care really works? Can you prove that your recommendations actually prevent disease and help people live longer?" My simple answer for the past 10 years has been a resounding *yes.* The secret lies in the health, or length, of your telomeres.

What's in a Telomere?

A telomere is a section of nucleotide sequences at the end of each of our chromosomes. (Nucleotides are organic molecules that form the basic structural unit of nucleic acids, such as DNA.) Each section is made up of more than 3,000 copies of the sequence TTAGGG. The repeated sequences protect the ends of chromosomes from unraveling, like aglets (the plastic end pieces) on a shoelace. Without them, our telomeres shorten and our cells die, leading to aging before our time.

In this chapter, I share with you pages of evidence that point a way forward. I include safe and effective strategies that show you how to live healthier, physically and mentally. Ultimately, we must also learn how to become more resilient to the ongoing effects of chronic health conditions. This pandemic will fade into the sunset in a few years, to a more benign virus, but we must learn from our collective experiences about the fragility of our health. As you'll recall from Chapter 1, most people who died from COVID-19 were either elderly or had preexisting conditions. It made them sitting ducks for the SARS-CoV-2 virus to attack them and cause significant sickness.

A Common Thread?

Objectively, researchers believe there may be a common thread that causes some patients to succumb to COVID-19. Short telomere length might serve as the biomarker, identifying patients who are more likely to die from the SARS-CoV-2 infection regardless of age. In particular, a low white blood cell count of lymphocytes, or lymphopenia, is another thread linking these patients. Scientists already know that short telomere length puts a limit on T-cell maturation into lymphocytes. Ultimately, this negatively impacts a person's ability to fight off an infection caused by SARS-CoV-2.[315]

Nobel Price–Winning Research

Telomere biology is a Nobel Prize–winning research field that simply didn't exist a generation ago. Over the past 30-plus years, scientists have worked to uncover the incredible predictive ability of telomeres to determine your biological age. Their work was so significant that in 2009 the Nobel Prize in Medicine was awarded jointly to three scientists, Drs. Elizabeth Blackburn, Carol Greider, and Jack Szostak, for discovering how telomeres protect our chromosomes and identifying the importance of the enzyme telomerase in this process.

Together, these three scientists solved a huge mystery in biology. How can our chromosomes be copied completely when our cells divide and how can they be protected from decaying and "dying"?

The scientists had to research the long, threadlike DNA molecules that carry our genes and are packed into 46 chromosomes to answer that question. It would soon be called the telomere portion of the chromosome.

Drs. Blackburn and Szostak discovered that a unique DNA sequence, called the telomere, protects our chromosomes from degrading. Then Drs. Greider and Blackburn discovered telomerase, which produces telomere DNA. When telomeres become shortened to a critical length, cells "age." On the other hand, if your body is producing enough telomerase, the length of your telomeres won't shorten (sometimes they can actually grow), and automatic cell death, what science calls cellular senescence, is delayed.

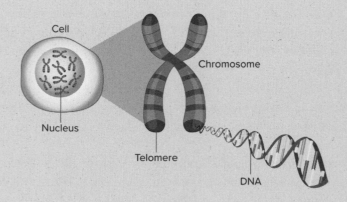

Cell

Nucleus

Chromosome

Telomere

DNA

Welcome to the Science of Antiaging and Telomere Biology

I'd like to look beyond the pandemic and focus on health strategies to live a longer and healthier life – not just free of COVID-19, but also from all chronic health conditions. Let's make the effort to not only improve our resiliency against physical and mental health issues, but, more importantly, slow the aging process by keeping our telomeres long and maybe even re-lengthening them.

The awarding of the Nobel Prize caused a surge of interest in the telomere field of medicine, and many more research groups are now working feverishly to determine which factors cause our telomeres to shorten before their time, and how telomeres can be re-lengthened. It will take some years to learn how to re-lengthen our telomeres safely. But today we know much more about why they age prematurely and how we can slow down our biological clocks.

This is why I'm so committed to speaking out about how important telomeres are in not dying young. Not only can telomeres predict your future health and your ability to fight viral infection, but they can also affect how long you'll live and how free of disease you'll be.

That's pretty powerful information. Today, with a simple test, you can learn how long your telomeres are. That one measure alone tells you how much your cells have aged and gives you an estimate of your true biological age. You should worry if your test shows that your cells have aged beyond your chronological or calendar age compared to people like you in age and gender. But don't run out to complete your bucket list on the basis of a telomere test. Instead, you should view your results as a chance to look at your life story so far and decide if you need to change a few things.

What's the real promise of telomeres? You can make the right lifestyle choices to ensure that your telomeres stay long and robust. And? You'll have as many years – and as many *good* years – as you possibly can.

Our desire to stay young and vibrant, live longer, and perform at our peak has been an ideal since we first walked the earth. The Greeks created the foundations of our modern Olympics, challenging a man's strength and speed and celebrating exemplary physical performance. Cleopatra of Egypt perfected the art of makeup. Indeed, ancient Egyptians' concerns with beauty and body care transcended gender lines. Women and men both used cosmetics and body oils. And for thousands of years, Chinese herbalists have created tinctures for vitality, mental acuity, and sexual prowess.

But I'll let you in on a secret: there's always been a Fountain of Youth – we just didn't know where to look for it. Now we do.

"Telomere maintenance is tied to the reasons why most people die . . . understanding [telomerase] may eventually be the basis for therapies to combat cancer, heart disease, and diabetes – perhaps even halt the ravages of age."[316]

— *Dr. Elizabeth Blackburn, Nobel Prize–winning scientist*

Living Your Full Lifespan Potential

Many scientists believe that genetics contributes only 20% to our longevity and that environmental factors determine the remaining 80%. This means we should be able to modify our lifestyle to improve our longevity.

Your biological parents gave you a set of genes, and these genes will play a major role in determining your lifespan. Your genes are housed in 46 chromosomes, and the tips of them – your telomeres – are also inherited. Genetics determines 80% of the variation in the length of your telomeres when you're born, but the role played by your parents in the variability of their length diminishes very quickly with time. In fact, that process starts right after you're conceived.

Scientists study identical twins to determine the roles that nature and nurture play in our development. You won't be surprised to learn that – although identical twins are born with the same number of telomere base pairs – researchers now know that environmental factors play the biggest role in telomere length after birth.[317, 318] In other words, telomere length in twins is the same at birth, but they shorten at different rates depending on the experiences and lifestyles of the individuals.

Initially, researchers believed that short telomeres were the *result* of aging – now we know telomere shortening is the *cause* of aging. So it follows that what you do with your life ultimately determines if you live out your genetic potential. It also can determine which diseases you'll contract as you age: the more you degrade your telomeres with poor lifestyle choices and physical and mental traumas, the sooner you'll be at risk for illness.

TELOMERE BURNOUT

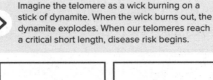

> Imagine the telomere as a wick burning on a stick of dynamite. When the wick burns out, the dynamite explodes. When our telomeres reach a critical short length, disease risk begins.

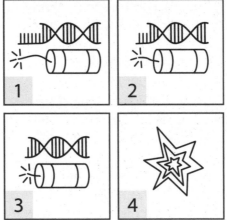

What's not as well-known is if the very ends of our DNA strands, like the aglets at the end of a shoelace, determine how long we'll live. Aglets, made of plastic or metal, stop your shoelaces from unraveling.

There's an important difference to understand in this simple comparison. When a shoelace does break down, we just buy another. But when a telomere can no longer do its job, the chromosomal cell it's protecting dies – and so does a part of you, aging your body and bringing you closer to chronic disease and possibly death. Telomeres are essentially your true biological clock, a major determinant of how long you will live and be healthy. People have often asked me, "So that's it? If I have too many short telomeres, I'm doomed?"

The answer is no.

Let's use a different analogy to help explain the real risk of telomere shortening. How quickly we wear away the treads on our car tires depends on a number of factors: how far we drive, the pressure in the tires, and how often and hard we slam on our brakes. Once our tires become bald, we can still drive on them, but they are less stable and reliable in wet weather. They can increase our risk of getting in an accident if we have a poor grip on the road. Ditto with short telomeres: they make our chromosomes less stable and put us at higher risk for developing abnormal cells and disease.

The Relationship Between Telomeres and Chronic Disease

We can change how our genetics play out over the course of our lives by slowing down the progression of telomere shortening and by re-lengthening our telomeres. Lifestyle changes play a role here, and we've covered many ways to improve your overall health and mental well-being in earlier chapters. This chapter reinforces the science of why it works.

Let's ponder what could happen if you ignore the science of telomeres. Just consider the relationship between telomeres and these chronic diseases:

Alzheimer's disease and dementia: Much shorter telomeres have been found among people who developed an aggressive decrease in brain function in both of these conditions.[319, 320]

Atherosclerosis (vascular disease): In atherosclerosis, which can lead to heart attacks and strokes, scientists have discovered that the blood vessel cells and smooth muscle cells next to areas of plaque formation have shorter telomeres than healthier counterparts in other areas of the body.[321] Another study found that shortened telomere pairs corresponded to a 300% increase in the risk of myocardial infarction and stroke.[322, 323] There's also a strong correlation between short telomeres and vascular dementia.[324]

Cancer: Many cancers involve chromosome rearrangement and mutations, and telomere shortening boosts the incidence of both.[325] This is why most cancers develop in older age.

Infections: Your immune system is highly sensitive to the shortening of telomeres. Its effectiveness depends on the ability of your white blood cells to proliferate during times of immunological stress. It turns out that if you have shorter white blood cell telomeres, you have an 800% higher mortality rate from infectious diseases.[326]

Liver cirrhosis: Hepatic (liver) cells have shorter telomeres. When the liver can't repair or reproduce its cells, it grows stiff and malfunctions.[327]

Osteoarthritis: In osteoarthritis and degenerative disk disease of the spine, cartilage cells have shorter telomeres. This results in a decreased regrowth of cartilage in joints,[328, 329] which results in less cartilage as we age and more grinding of bone on bone, causing pain and inflammation in our joints.

Osteoporosis (bone-thinning disease): Bone cells called osteoclasts remodel our bones, and other bone cells called osteoblasts rebuild our bones. In osteoporosis, the osteoclasts keep remodeling, but osteoblastic cells fail to rebuild. Science has discovered a link between the incidence of osteoporosis and shorter telomeres in osteoblast cells.[330, 331]

Wrinkles: Although not life-threatening, wrinkles are a condition we all experience as we age. But why are some people more wrinkled than others? Short telomeres have been linked to the malfunctioning of the basal cell layer, which causes a thinning of skin and age spots.[332]

Preventive Care Outperforms Disease Management

I've said it many times in many public forums over the years: our health system needs to change from managing disease to preventing disease before it starts. And knowing how telomeres fit into the preventive health mix is definitely an antiaging breakthrough. As of now, it's possible to slow our telomere shortening by changing our lifestyle to reduce inflammation, glycation, and oxidative stress and to improve the balance of our hormones.

But these steps aren't as powerful as actually lengthening our telomeres as we age. Just imagine the possibilities for our health if we could do that. Well, that day is not far off. Scientists around the globe are working to discover how to activate the enzyme telomerase. The secret to re-lengthening our telomeres may lie in our ability to alter the activity of this enzyme.

Telomerase is an enzyme that protects our DNA from unraveling and mutating. If we could get it to work on our behalf, we could be free of many of the diseases that kill us now and live much longer by:

Reducing inflammation: Inflammation is a protective response by the body to rid itself of the harm caused by pathogens (such as bacteria and viruses) and irritants. In this process of repair and healing, tissues can be damaged, which leads to damaged organs and disease.

Preventing oxidative stress: Oxidation occurs when an oxygen molecule binds to a substance such as organ tissue and causes a change in its chemical structure, thereby creating an unstable, destructive molecule known as a free radical. Long-term damage by these molecules can lead to DNA damage, loss of cellular energy, and – ultimately – cell death.

Avoiding glycation: Glycation weakens your body's biomolecules. It binds sugar molecules to lipid or protein molecules inside your body's tissues. This causes your organs, such as your kidneys and even your eyes, to malfunction. Glycation is implicated in many age-related chronic diseases, such as cardiovascular diseases, Alzheimer's disease, and cancer.

By measuring and managing variables such as inflammation, oxidation, and glycation, you can slow down the destruction of your telomeres. Of course, each of us is different and will respond to certain techniques better than others. Thankfully, it's possible to calculate the rate of this shortening using a simple blood test that measures your telomere length, so you can determine if any of the interventions and treatments I have recommended in this book are working for you. Welcome to personalized antiaging medicine.

In theory, it may be possible to induce the human telomerase gene to produce telomerase. Having the ability to prevent cells from aging would forever change the landscape of medicine – and, really, life as we know it. This sounds dramatic, and it is. Later in this chapter, I also discuss the future of stem cells and how stem cell therapy may change our aging trajectory.

Age-Proof Your Lifestyle

Small Choices Make a Big Difference

Your telomeres are telling on you; it's time to age-proof your lifestyle. We've known for years that not getting enough sleep, not exercising enough, and using recreational drugs can impact your health in a bad way.

But now we can see the effects of these factors in the length of our telomeres.

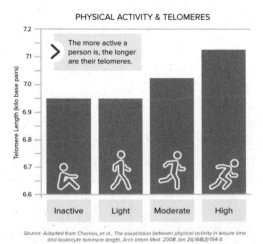

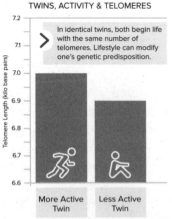

PHYSICAL ACTIVITY & TELOMERES

The more active a person is, the longer are their telomeres.

Source: Adapted from Cherkas, et al., The association between physical activity in leisure time and leukocyte telomere length, Arch Intern Med. 2008 Jon 28;168(2):154-8

TWINS, ACTIVITY & TELOMERES

In identical twins, both begin life with the same number of telomeres. Lifestyle can modify one's genetic predisposition.

Source: Adapted from Cherkas, et al., The association between physical activity in leisure time and leukocyte telomere length, Arch Intern Med. 2008;168(2):154-158

SLEEP

Now that we know there's a relationship between sleep and chronic disease, let's identify the biological link. Research shows a correlation between the quantity and quality of our sleep and the length of our telomeres.

A study involving 10,000 people showed a direct relationship between telomere length and sleep duration. The men in the study who reported they were getting more than 7 hours of sleep each night had telomeres that were longer than those men sleeping fewer than 5 hours a night. In fact, the "short sleepers" had telomeres that were 6% shorter on average.[333]

Another study of 245 women showed similar results – women with chronically poor sleep quality displayed telomeres that were shorter.[334]

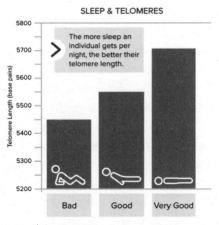

Source: Adapted from Shorter leukocyte telomere length in midlife women with poor sleep quality, by Prather AA, Puterman E, Lin J, O'Donovan A, Krauss J, Tomiyama AJ, Epel ES, and Blackburn EH. J Aging Res. 2011;2011:721390

Sleep Apnea and Telomere Length

We know that sleep apnea is a sleep disorder and is not historically linked to lifestyle. But we also know that people who are obese are more likely to develop sleep apnea. It is characterized by abnormal pauses in breathing; these breaks can be as short as 10 seconds or they can last minutes, and they can happen as many as 30 times or more an hour. As a result of this abnormal breathing behavior, low oxygenation in the body results.

A group of French scientists showed that telomere length was much shorter in patients with OSAS (obstructive sleep apnea syndrome).[335] If left untreated, conditions that disrupt sleep, such as sleep apnea, can cause heart disease, pulmonary hypertension, and high blood pressure, and this has also been linked to type 2 diabetes.

ALCOHOL AND SMOKING

You don't need to see your telomeres under a microscope to know that smoking and drinking don't mix with good health. But using the two most common legalized recreational drugs in the world is one surefire way to burn up your telomeres.

Let's start with alcohol. We've come a long way with curbing drinking and driving, and the combination of drinking and health deserves just as much attention. Heavy alcohol consumption has been linked to increased oxidation stress and inflammation (and we know how those two things can speed up telomere shortening) as well as to cancer risk.

Studies show that your telomere length can decrease in relation to the number of alcoholic drinks consumed in a day. People who drank more than four drinks a day showed telomeres that were half the length of those enjoying less than one drink a day.[336]

Personally, I don't think that even one drink a day is safe, at least from a cancer perspective. Although there is data to suggest that a drink or two a day is cardio-protective, the opposite is true for cancer. In fact, your risk of mouth and pharynx cancer goes up by 17% if you consume just one drink a day; breast cancer risk in women goes up by 5%. Worldwide, every year, over 2 million deaths are linked to alcohol, according to a report in the *Annals of Oncology* – and the same report attributes 3.6% of all cancers to drinking alcohol.[337] Dr. Thomas Sellers at the Mayo Clinic found that women who are daily drinkers and had close relatives with breast cancer doubled their risk of developing breast cancer compared to women who also had close relatives with breast cancer but never consumed alcohol.[338] So, is that drink really worth it?

To bring the message home, a recent Harvard study showed a dose-dependent risk of the number of alcoholic drinks and the risk of developing breast cancer. Women who drank three to six drinks a week increased their breast cancer risk by 15%, and those who drank an average of two drinks a day increased their risk by 51%.[339]

If developing cancer does not scare you but dying of COVID-19 does, then let me give you another data point. Many of my patients enjoy half a bottle of wine each night. We routinely see low white blood cell counts in heavy drinkers, and once alcohol consumption is reduced, the cell count bounces back. We do know that alcohol blunts the production of CD4 T cells,[340] which, as noted earlier, is an important natural antiviral.

And if you light up a cigarette or cigar with your drink, you're just asking for trouble. Watch as that cigarette burns down. It's the perfect metaphor for telomere shortening – shown at high speed. Simply put, tobacco smoking shortens telomeres faster than not smoking, as shown by Ana Valdes and others in a 2005 study.[341]

For those who say they are only a social smoker, data suggests that any smoker, regardless of whether they drink alcohol or not, has shorter telomeres. Like alcohol, there is no "safe dose" of tobacco smoking when it relates to telomere health, but there is a dose-dependent effect. The more cigarettes you smoke in your life, the shorter your telomeres will become.

There is a lot of information to support this claim. First, we know smoking can cause inflammation throughout the body; second, it's well-known that it also causes oxidative stress.[342] These two processes have been well discussed in earlier chapters, and we know that inflammation and oxidation are two of the four big health enemies in telomere health, along with glycation and hormone imbalance.

Mental Health Affects Physical Health: A Proven Relationship

Finally, we have proof of what medicine has long suspected: our mental health can drive our physical health. Stress leads to shorter telomeres. We finally have biological proof that chronic physical diseases are intertwined with a lack of mental well-being.

Many small studies have found that people who have been suffering from depression for long periods of time have shorter telomeres. In fact, the rate appears to be in line with the total number of days a person is depressed over their lifetime. Oxidative stress and inflammation seem to be related to this process.[343] In other words, our physical maladies are related in some way to our mental ones.

A groundbreaking study in 2004 highlights the link between stress and the rate of telomere shortening. The researchers looked at the telomere lengths of mothers who were responsible for the care of their chronically ill children.

The longer a mother spent time as the main caregiver of a child affected by a serious disorder, the shorter her telomeres were compared to mothers caring for children who were generally healthy. They also found that mothers who felt a sense of control over their lives had longer telomeres than mothers who felt their lives were more stressed. Quantified, the "most stressed" mothers exhibited telomere shortening equal to at least 10 years of aging.[344] This means that this stress could shorten their lives by 10 years.

Many researchers have strengthened the cause-and-effect connection between chronic stress and shorter telomere length since that study was published. In fact, they have found chronic stress may indeed *cause* our

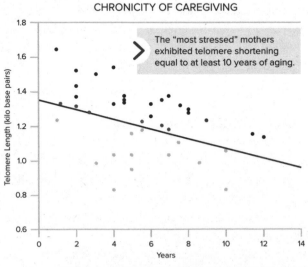

CHRONICITY OF CAREGIVING

The "most stressed" mothers exhibited telomere shortening equal to at least 10 years of aging.

Source: Epel, et al., Proc Natl Acad Sci USA. 2004 Dec 7;101(49):17312-5

telomeres to shorten (not just that there is a *link*). A 2011 study showed that this causal effect appears to start at a very early age – in childhood and perhaps even before a child is born. It found that young healthy adults of mothers who experienced relatively stress-free pregnancies display longer telomeres than their peers whose mothers experienced severe stress while pregnant – such as the stress that happens after the death of a close family member.[345]

> "We now know that stress seeps into the cell and changes hundreds of biological processes, including the rate of aging. . . . Telomeres are the clock or pacemaker of the cell's life. . . . It appears our cells are listening to our suffering and eavesdropping in on our thoughts. The implications [of this mind–cell relationship] are vast."[346]
>
> — *Dr. Elissa Epel, PhD, Dept. of Psychiatry, UCSF*

The Power of Telomerase

The world of medicine believes that telomeres are stable structures that shorten slowly over many years. Some scientists had assumed that our telomere length does not change over a period of months. However, some small studies have found the opposite to be true. Telomerase activity can be increased and responsive to certain lifestyle and mindset changes quite quickly.

Definition: Telomerase

Telomerase is an enzyme that carries its own ribonucleic acid (RNA) template for DNA synthesis. In the language of science, it is what is known as a reverse transcriptase – that is to say, it is an enzyme that catalyzes the formation of RNA from a DNA template during cell replication, or transcription. This enzyme, when activated, can re-lengthen telomeres.

In an uncontrolled study, celebrated physician Dr. Dean Ornish oversaw an intensive lifestyle modification program for men with prostate cancer. Those who followed a plant-based diet (high in fruits, vegetables, and unrefined grains, and low in fat and refined carbohydrates), increased their physical activity, and used stress-reduction techniques (such as yoga, meditation, and social support) saw their telomerase activity increase by 30% over 3 months.[347]

In another study, overweight women followed a program that involved stress reduction and mindful eating. The study found that their telomerase activity increased by 18% in a treatment group compared to the control group.[348] What's more, those women who showed the largest decreases in psychological distress, cortisol, and glucose also showed the greatest increases in telomerase activity. (Recall that lower cortisol levels leads to lower insulin, which stabilizes blood glucose levels. When this occurs, your aging processes are reduced.) Please see below for more information on how meditation can boost telomerase activity.

In a study of dementia caregivers (men and women who care for patients with dementia), a group practicing meditation showed more telomerase activity – 43% more – compared to a relaxation control group.[349]

Can We Activate Telomerase?

In theory, it may be possible to induce the human telomerase gene to produce telomerase (recall this enzyme can repair telomeres). As it stands now, each human cell divides a certain number of times before entering a nondividing state called replicative senescence. The number of times a cell can divide is called a cell's Hayflick limit. Different kinds of cells have different Hayflick limits (skin cells in a petri dish, for example, can divide approximately 50 times before they stop dividing). When enough of an organ's cells have died, the organ begins to function inefficiently. This leads to organ failure, which eventually can lead to the organism dying. We now know that this mechanism of telomere shortening causes cellular senescence, or cell death. However, cancer cells divide indefinitely, defying this limit. Today we know this is caused by the continuous activation of telomerase within unhealthy cells.

So it seems that if we could kick-start our body's production of telomerase, we could extend the limits of all our healthy cells and reap the benefits of robust telomeres indefinitely. That would change the nature of medicine completely – but it's a very big "if."

How Does Meditation Prompt Telomerase Activity?

The effects of stress on telomere shortening may build up over time rather than be caused by a single event, although how severe the stressor is and the perceived threat also play roles. Therefore, to prevent our telomeres from prematurely shortening, we must focus on how we can improve our health and mental well-being – even after COVID lockdowns – so we can become more resilient against health risk factors.

A more definitive study investigated the effects of a 3-month meditation retreat on telomerase activity and two major stress contributors: the perceived control of one's life (associated with decreased stress) and neuroticism (associated with increased subjective distress). Thirty retreat subjects meditated for 3 months for 6 hours each day. The researchers looked at mindfulness as one quality cultivated by meditative practice and at another quality developed during meditative practice. This latter quality hasn't been studied in depth – a shift in intentions and priorities, away from boosting your "hedonic" pleasure (superficial well-being) to making a deeper "purpose in life" more clear. Telomerase activity was significantly greater in retreat participants than in controls at the end of the retreat. The retreat group also displayed increases in perceived control. Mindfulness and purpose in life were also greater. This study was one of the first to link meditation and positive psychological change with telomerase activity.[350]

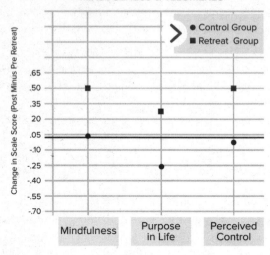

Based on telomere and telomerase biology, to live a longer, healthier life, we should manage our lifestyle by:

- Eating healthy and balanced meals
- Sleeping enough and sleeping well
- Exercising in many ways
- Including mindfulness practices
- And, last but not least, having a strong life purpose

Long Haulers of COVID-19

We know that some people experience a type of post-viral syndrome after becoming sick with COVID-19. These patients are now called long haulers. The incidence ranges from 10% to 80%, depending on which study you review. The most common physical symptoms are fatigue and body aches, shortness of breath, difficulty concentrating, inability to exercise, headache, and difficulty sleeping. Anxiety is an ongoing mental health concern for some long haulers.

The post-viral reaction not only strikes those who have been very sick and required ICU intubation care, but also those who have been weathering the infection at home.

In a group of 143 Italian patients ages 19 to 84, 125 (87%) still experienced COVID-19–related symptoms an average of 2 months after their first symptom was noted. All the patients had been hospitalized, with their stays averaging about 2 weeks, and 80% hadn't received any form of ventilation.[351] In May 2020, a French hospital survey of 30 patients per week found that men (average age 40) experienced a post-viral reaction four times more than women.

> "Anecdotally, there's no question that there are a considerable number of individuals who have a post-viral syndrome that really, in many respects, can incapacitate them for weeks and weeks following so-called recovery and clearing of the virus."[352]
> — *Anthony Fauci, MD, director of the National Institute of Allergy and Infectious Diseases*

Multisystem Organ Failure

Multisystem organ failure (MSOF) occurs in some COVID-19 patients. In addition to lung damage, some people experience damage to the heart, liver, kidney, brain, and hematological system. MSOF is often triggered by a severe inflammatory reaction caused by an overactive immune system, and this is followed by a hyper-coagulation event leading to blood clots in some organs.[353]

Kidney Problems

Once an organ is damaged and can't be salvaged, patients often hope for an organ transplant. Several longitudinal studies showed that some people who experienced severe cases of COVID-19 are showing signs of kidney damage, even if they had no previous underlying kidney problems.[354] Up to 30% of patients hospitalized with COVID-19 in China and New York developed moderate or severe kidney injury.[355] Some may need dialysis, and this is often a precursor to requiring a kidney transplant.

In April 2021, my training hospital, University Health Network, performed the world's first double-lung transplant on a recovered COVID-19 patient who was otherwise healthy.[356]

This begs the question: How many of these types of organ transplants will be required by long haulers? Unfortunately, the need for donor organs is far greater than the supply available. Therefore, we must look at other technologies.

Canadian Organ Donations

Canadian organ donor facts from the David Foster Foundation:

- In 2020, registration was down 39% due to the COVID-19 pandemic.
- More than 4,500 Canadians are currently waiting for a lifesaving organ transplant, and each year approximately 1,600 people are added to the list.
- Of those on the wait-list, approximately five people die each week, or one death every 30 hours, all of which could have been avoided.
- One organ donor can save up to eight lives and improve the quality of life for up to 75 people.

Visit www.LiveOn.ca to find out how to become an organ donor in your Canadian province or territory, or https://unos.org/transplant in the United States.

The Future of Stem Cells to Grow New Organs

In the early 1960s, two University of Toronto researchers, physicist James Till and biologist Ernest McCulloch, discovered stem cells in the human body. Today, their work allows us to do lifesaving bone marrow transplants for blood diseases such as leukemia and aplastic anemia. Donor stem cells, which can sometimes come from the patient themselves, can be put into "sick" bone marrow and grow as a new blood system for the recipient.

These days, stem cell therapy, also known as regenerative medicine, is being used in more than just bone marrow transplantation. Scientists are now working with stem cells and their derivatives to treat other diseased, dysfunctional, or injured tissues. Stem cells can be manipulated to become specialized stem cells, such as skin, pancreatic, kidney, and heart tissues. Biological labs are now growing organs with the hope of one day transplanting them into humans. The most studied stem cell research areas include:

- Macular degeneration
- Neurological conditions (such as Parkinson's disease and Huntington's disease)
- Diabetes
- Spinal cord injury
- Myocardial infarction
- Multiple sclerosis
- Leukemia
- Cartilage/tendon injuries
- Skin burns
- Damaged cornea

Two types of stem cells are used for scientific research:

1. **Adult or tissue stem cells.** As the name suggests, these are mature cells that have already developed into a specific type of tissue. So, for example, we can harvest liver cells to regenerate liver tissue, and muscle stem cells to regenerate muscle fibers. We can't use liver cells to develop muscles fibers (and vice versa), because these stem cells are already so specialized.
2. **Embryonic stem cells.** This type of stem cell is deemed pluripotent, meaning these cells can develop into thousands of tissue types. In other words, they are master-builder cells and can become skin cells, brain cells, muscle cells, liver cells, and more.

In the early days of stem cell research, some felt that taking embryonic cord blood from aborted fetuses was an unacceptable way to harvest stem cells. Today, stem cells can also be harvested from umbilical cord blood after delivery and from some types of adult tissues with the help of new scientific technologies still under development. We call these kinds of cells induced pluripotent stem (iPS) cells, and they were first discovered in 2006 by Shinya Yamanaka. He won a Nobel Prize in 2012 for his work on reprogramming adult cells to exist in an embryonic-like state.[357]

iPS Cell Lines for Personalized Medicine

Cell-based treatments are most effective with our youngest cells. This makes it important to collect and preserve the best cells today. For example, you can stop the aging process of the cells in your follicle by plucking your hair and cryopreserving the follicle at $-320°F$ ($-196°C$). This ensures that the cells stay healthy and viable for future use, waiting for science to catch up. The regrowth of hair and skin cells for cosmetic antiaging is just a few years away. And research is well underway to transplant heart cells rather than implant a mechanical pacemaker to keep a steady cardiac rhythm.

I have frozen my own hair follicles, and also those of my son, at Acorn Biolabs (www.acorn.me). Soon I may want some new skin cells to refresh my facial features, if I'm looking for an alternative to skin fillers and neurotoxins like Botox. The process would involve injecting iPS cells derived from my hair follicle cells into my skin, which would cause my skin cells to grow younger cells.

Certainly, by the time my son is old, and if for some reason he needs an organ transplant, he may be able to grow his own organ at a biological age of 18 years, the age when I froze his hair follicle.

Generating iPS cell lines requires time and lab resources. The cells require genetic manipulation and could theoretically mutate from their natural stem cell lines. Therefore, cells must be carefully tested to make sure they did not mutate negatively during processing. Given the significant opportunity to treat and repair so many organs and reverse end-stage chronic disease, this kind of research is well underway, despite the huge challenges.

We must lean into using our own iPS cell lines, which will elevate personalized medicine to a new level. Let's continue to push forward with personalized medicine and use our cells to develop therapies just for ourselves. By growing tissues and organs, we can treat trauma, chronic illness, and aging conditions – and even the organ damage caused by COVID-19.

CHAPTER 12

Your Antiaging Checklist

Every day, you need to tap into what drives you to want to live and to stay healthy, happy, and personally fulfilled. This will always be a work in progress. So calibrate yourself, and recalibrate often by measuring your vital signs and monitoring your health biomarkers. Do the lifestyle work you need to do. Upgrade yourself physically, mentally, and spiritually. It is possible to live a long and healthy life, but it takes not only physical work but also mindful work.

10 Categories of Tests to complete annually

Note: Some of the tests in this list may not have been explicitly described in this book but are informative to a specialized antiaging, integrative medicine health practitioner.

1. **Vital signs**
    *   Weight
    *   Blood pressure
    *   Heart rate
    *   Waist circumference
    *   Lung – aerobic capacity (VO2)
    *   Percentage body fat

- Percentage visceral fat
- Percentage muscle mass

2. **Basic routine labs**
   - Glucose, HgbA1c
   - Cholesterol (total and triglycerides)
   - Organ system function for:
     - Liver
       - AST (aspartate transaminase)
       - ALT (alanine transferase)
       - ALP (alkaline phosphatase)
       - GGT (gamma-glutamyl transpeptidase)
     - Kidney
       - Creatinine
       - Glomerular filtration rate
       - Urinalysis
   - Hematology
     - Hemoglobin (red blood cells)
     - White blood cells
     - Platelet count

3. **Hormones**
   - Estrogens (estradiol, estriol, estrone)
   - Progesterone
   - Testosterone
   - Dehydroepiandrosterone (DHEA)
   - Thyroid function (TSH – thyroid stimulating hormone, T4, and T3)
   - Insulin
   - Growth hormone
   - Cortisol
   - Melatonin

4. **Mental health labs**
   - Serotonin
   - GABA

- Dopamine
- Epinephrine/norepinephrine

5. **Nutrient markers**
   - Vitamins
   - Minerals
   - Amino acids
   - Fatty acids
   - Organic acids

6. **Toxin panel**
   - Mercury
   - Lead
   - Arsenic
   - Cadmium

7. **Inflammation panel**
   - C-reactive protein
   - Homocysteine
   - Arachidonic acid
   - Prostaglandins
   - Interleukins
   - Omega fatty acids

8. **Oxidation panel**
   - Vitamin C
   - Coenzyme Q_{10}
   - Superoxide dismutase
   - Lipid peroxidase
   - Glutathione peroxidase

9. **Antibodies testing**
   - Food sensitivities
   - Environmental sensitivities
   - COVID-19
     - Nucleocapsid (N protein)

- Spike (S protein)
- Pseudo Nutralization
- Avidity

10. Genetics tests
- Telomere test
  - Average length
  - Percentage short telomeres

11. General
- Pharmacogenetics
- Nutrigenomics
- Disease risk – population genetics
- Mutations

10 Lifestyle Actions

Here is my top 10 list of things to improve your health resiliency and prevent your telomeres from shortening prematurely.

1. **Lose weight.** As we've discussed, people who are overweight are at greater risk for many health conditions, and their shorter telomeres reflect this at a cellular level.

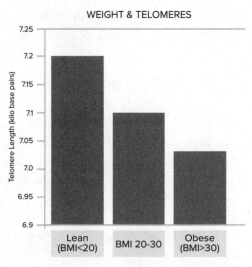

WEIGHT & TELOMERES

Source: Valdes, et al., Lancet. 2005 Aug 20-26;366(9486):662-4

2. **Exercise.** It's never too late to start exercising. Your telomere length can improve at any age. Whether you walk or run, swim or do tai chi, kickbox or bicycle, it's important to be active at least 30 minutes every day.

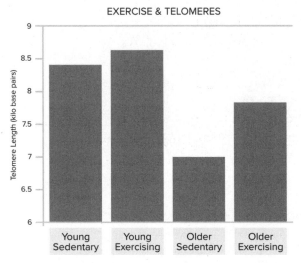

EXERCISE & TELOMERES

Source: LaRocca, et al., Mech Ageing Dev. 2010 Feb;131(2):165-7

3. **Reduce alcohol consumption.** There is a stark difference in telomere length between alcoholics and social drinkers or nondrinkers.

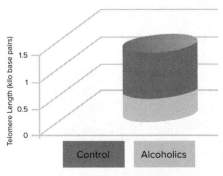
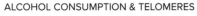

ALCOHOL CONSUMPTION & TELOMERES

Source: Sofia Pavanello et al., International Journal of cancer,
Int. J. Cancer: 129, 983-992 (2011) VC 2011 UICC

4. **Do not smoke.** Need we say more about this topic? Here's more proof why you should quit. As you can see, smoking shortens telomeres prematurely, and if you keep smoking, telomeres will keep shortening.

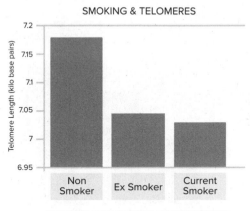

SMOKING & TELOMERES

Source: Valdes, et al., Lancet. 2005 Aug 20-26;366(9486):662-4

5. **Increase your consumption of fish.** Doing so will improve your level of omega fatty acids, nature's anti-inflammatory. The more fish you eat, the less your telomeres shorten.

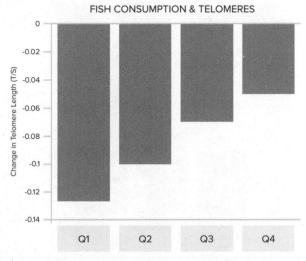

FISH CONSUMPTION & TELOMERES

Source: Farzaneh-Far, et al., JAMA. 2010 Jan 20;303(3):250-7

6. **Get in the sun.** Vitamin D, the sunshine vitamin, is a potent fat-soluble antioxidant that has anti-inflammatory effects.

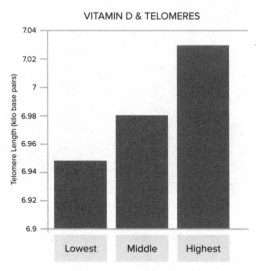

Source: Richards, et al., Am J Clin Nutr. 2007 Nov;86(5):1420-5

7. **Sleep more.** Improve both the quantity and quality of your sleep.

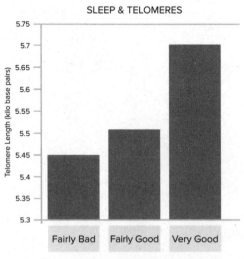

Source: Arica A. Prather, Elizabteh H. Blackburn, et al., Journal of aging research, volume 2011 (2011)

8. **Treat, manage, and resolve mental health conditions.** Many people suffer in silence. The sooner it resolves, the slower your telomeres unravel.

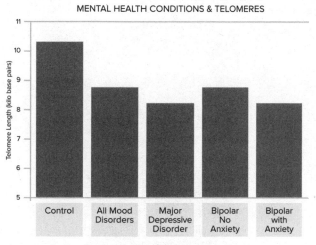

MENTAL HEALTH CONDITIONS & TELOMERES

Source: Simon, et al., Biol Psychiatry. 2006 Sep 1;60(5):432-5

9. **Be happy.** It's important to have a positive outlook and believe that we will all get through this pandemic – not only stronger physically and mentally than when we went into it, but perhaps even happier as we set new goals for living a more purposeful life.

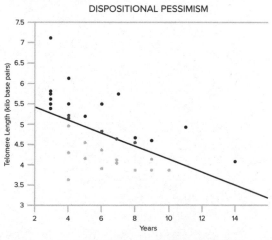

DISPOSITIONAL PESSIMISM

Source: O<Donovan, et al., Brain Behav Immun, 2009 May;23(4):446-9

10. **Meditate.** This is a type of mindfulness practice that many people have now adopted as a way to relieve stress. We know that those who regularly practice meditation have longer telomeres than those who do not. Meditation works by activating the enzyme telomerase.

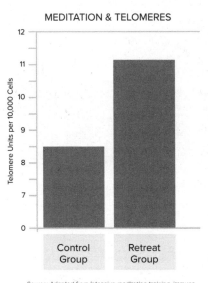

MEDITATION & TELOMERES

Source: Adapted from Intensive meditation training, immune cell telomerase activity, and psychological mediators. T.L. Jacobs et al., #2010 Elsevier Ltd.

Conclusion

Congratulations! You're at the final section of this book. Thank you for staying focused along with me. This book is your manifesto, a kind of companion for living a longer and healthier life. COVID-19 has taught us a lot of things, not least of which is that we are all susceptible to sudden illness. Our vulnerabilities have been exposed on a number of levels, most especially when it comes to our health and well-being. SARS-CoV-2 has demonstrated just how lethal a disease it is, and without our fitness and health, it had the ability to deal a blow that would leave many of us severely ill.

Postmortem

During the course of the pandemic, I have been invited onto a number of news programs to talk about COVID-19 topics. And in May 2021, Amanda Lang, a national business journalist, interviewed me on BNN Bloomberg (Canada). She ended our conversation by asking me what "we" should have done differently. We both chuckled cynically, and I offered up two suggestions in the interest of time. One was to manage the timing of lockdowns and reopenings more strategically, and the other was for Canada to position itself as a manufacturer of vaccines and to be nationally self-sustainable. I could have gone on for many more minutes.

Some countries managed to gain control of the pandemic better than others. Unfortunately, North America and Europe did not make the "in control" list. In fact, the World Health Organization (WHO) concluded in a report published in March 2021 that COVID-19 was, in fact, "a preventable disaster."[358]

Here's a brief summary of what I believe contributed to how we found ourselves ill-prepared for what turned out to be a pandemic of epic proportions.

- The virus was new and far more contagious than the Chinese government and the WHO were willing to admit. (In the spirit of lost opportunities, the WHO described February 2020 as the "lost" month – a squandered opportunity to contain the virus).
- SARS-CoV-2 turned out to be a respiratory virus and there were far more asymptomatic spreaders than we first thought (approximately 40% to 60% are carriers).
- There was a global shortage of PPE and China was a leading supplier for the world when the pandemic began.
- The WHO failed to lead, and governments around the world created narratives to fit their own political agendas. Some were also unable or unwilling to get their citizens to do simple things like put on a mask.
- Borders remained open for far too long, and people moved around the globe spreading the virus for months before travel bans were put into place.
- Messaging from scientists about the virus's danger and the need for PPE and social distancing was confusing and changed as the science evolved.
- People became exhausted by the mixed messaging. This problem was exacerbated by politicians who determined how to share the scientific information and at times chose to even spread misinformation too.

The postmortem is still being written. Herd immunity (when the virus stops spreading because there are no longer enough hosts to ensure its survival) may remain elusive. The precise immunity level to achieve herd immunity is an unknown at this time. Some scientists have placed the threshold at 60% to 70% of the population gaining immunity, either through vaccinations or from past exposure to the virus.[359]

Anthony Fauci, director of the National Institute of Allergy and Infectious Diseases, admitted he has been incrementally raising his herd-immunity estimate over time as the true number may not be welcomed by the public and politicians alike. He believes that a rate of 90% will be required. This percentage is the same immunity level required to stop a measles outbreak. (Measles is highly contagious, not dissimilar to some COVID-19 variant strains.)[360]

> "We'll never achieve herd immunity, but that does in no way diminish the value of vaccines."
> — *Dr. Paul Hunter, professor of Medicine,*
> *University of East Anglia, England*

Dr. Hunter does not believe that the world will achieve herd immunity given the reality of vaccine hesitancy and the development of highly contagious new COVID-19 variants.[361]

Because of the low probability of achieving herd immunity worldwide in the near future, I believe the world is about to enter the endemic phase of this epidemic. The SARS-CoV-2 virus will likely remain with us well into 2022/23. In the meantime, countries still have enormous hurdles to overcome with vaccination manufacturing, distribution and administration, and containment of the variant strains. The precise execution of a worldwide COVID-19 vaccine rollout will ultimately determine the recovery of global economies and small businesses everywhere.

Definition: Endemic

"An endemic disease can always be found amongst a specific community or group of people living in one particular area of the world."[362]

— Oxford Reference

We are not safe until all of us are safe. It's a mantra I have repeated a number of times. So long as we have transmission, we will have mutations. If we see significant variants of concern and we experience vaccine escape, we will need more and more vaccine boosters for years to come. The pandemic, in other words, will morph into an endemic.

An Evolving Endemic

Indeed, many scientists believe the SARS-CoV-2 virus is here to stay and that we will live with it for a long time to come. A February 2021 *Nature* magazine survey of global scientists reported that 90% of respondents believed this coronavirus would evolve into an endemic, meaning the virus will continue to circulate in pockets of the global population for many years.

> "Eradicating this virus right now from the world is a lot like trying to plan the construction of a stepping-stone pathway to the moon. It's unrealistic."[363]
>
> — *Michael Osterholm, epidemiologist at the University of Minnesota in Minneapolis*

The good news is, more than one-third of the respondents in the *Nature* magazine report say they thought that it might be possible to eliminate SARS-CoV-2 from some regions while it continued to circulate in others at one given point in time.[364]

These same scientists say we have every reason to believe this coronavirus will become less dangerous as it evolves. Influenza and some coronaviruses are already endemic. It's why we have annual flu shots to boost our immune system to fight off infection, something we are likely to see with COVID-19. We have thankfully not needed lockdowns to manage our flu seasons so far.

And for physicians like me, the 2020/21 flu season did not materialize. We didn't see many people with colds and flus. Data shows that the incidence of flu cases was low, thanks to all the public health measures in place. It proves that more handwashing and the occasional use of masks when we have a cold or flu would not hurt.[365]

As vaccines become more available and people get their shots, we will reduce the hospitalization and death rates, something we are already beginning to see. Between December 2020 and May 2021, many territories, including the United Kingdom and the United States, have been vaccinating their citizens quite aggressively. Both have seen dramatic improvements in their COVID-19 statistics.[366, 367]

Thankfully, the SARS-CoV-2 virus seems so far to be evolving much slower than the influenza virus. This helps to reduce vaccine escape, when a virus can evade our immune defenses. It's why, in the next few years, in an attempt to create a safer world, we will likely need to get booster vaccinations against variant strains for SARS-CoV-2, just like annual flu shots against influenza.

The Microtraumas of the Pandemic

By definition, a pandemic is already a global event. No one on planet Earth has been spared. In 2020/21, personal freedoms were impacted by public health mandates, and our lives were forever changed and scarred by COVID-19 illnesses and death. On the surface, this pandemic can appear to be one huge traumatic experience, but in fact, it has been an accumulation of numerous microtraumas.

In earlier chapters, I discussed the topic of stress and its impact on our health. With COVID-19, we have encountered multiple microtraumas for over a year. Every few days, there was something new. We were told the virus was contagious, but it was unclear how we should keep ourselves and our loved ones safe from getting COVID-19. There was a rush to get cleaning materials and masks – and, yes, toilet paper too. Our work and home lives changed in a matter of weeks, and still today, we are juggling everything from remaining gainfully employed to looking after our financial security and our children's schooling, not to mention our loss of a social life.

COVID-19 Events

Here's a short list of COVID-19 events that have caused all of us to feel vulnerable and helpless:

- Discovering there is a lethal virus circulating the world and later learning that it is in our workplace, community, or home

- Being told initially that the virus was transported by air droplets, only to be informed later that it is a virus that is transmitted through respiration, and that it and can travel across a closed space very easily
- Navigating the changing recommendations around masking – being told early on that a cloth mask was adequate, and later being told that a medical-grade mask is needed – and double masking was better
- Discovering a global shortage of masks, hand sanitizers, and cleaning materials
- Finding short supplies of PPE, respirators, and treatment medications in hospitals
- Dealing with the lagging treatments to eradicate COVID-19
- Shifting to home school and working virtually
- Experiencing increased job insecurity, leading to financial and food insecurity
- Navigating shut regional and international borders
- Learning that vulnerable communities are isolated from support or experiencing isolation
- Experiencing ongoing concerns of vaccination procurement, access, safety, and efficacy
- Experiencing fears and anxiety about returning to work in person

Even if a person is exposed to only one traumatic event, it's often a stressful time. And it becomes far more stressful when traumatic experiences are recurrent and ongoing. How someone experiences and copes with a single trauma will determine how long its effects will last. Indeed, the more frequently we experience traumatic events in our lives, and how well we manage each occurrence, will define many of our longer-term health issues.

These traumas can impact our neurobiological composition as well. In other words, the mind–body connection will determine our ability to cope, feel trust, manage cognitive processes, and regulate our behavior. Experiencing a series of prolonged, unpredictable, and uncontrollable events caused by the COVID-19 pandemic can lead to traumatic changes that stress our body and mind.

There are three components to a traumatic event. They are often referred to as the three Es of trauma: event, experience, and effect.

Individual trauma results from an event, a series of events, or a set of circumstances that is experienced by an individual as physically or emotionally harmful or life-threatening, and that has lasting adverse effects on the individual's functioning and mental, physical, social, emotional, or spiritual well-being.[368]

Source: Substance Abuse and Mental Health
Services Administration (SAMHSA)

In my view, the impact of these microtraumas is the reason why many of us are not able to "get on" with it.

In October 2020, the American Psychological Association (APA) warned about the impact of stressful events on our long-term physical and mental health. And moving forward, we will be fighting more than just the COVID-19 endemic. The healthcare system will inevitably experience an epidemic of fewer healthy people who are physically or mentally well.

An APA survey conducted in late February 2021 found that people's physical health has already declined. APA believes this is a result of their inability to cope in healthy ways with the stresses of the pandemic. Many people continue to struggle with maintaining a desired healthy weight and getting enough quality sleep, and many have turned to alcohol as a coping mechanism. The groups at higher risk continue to be parents, essential workers, young people, and people of color.[369]

Not surprisingly, but problematic for primary care health providers, the APA survey confirmed many people had delayed their medical appointments. Physicians, including me, believe that many people are now going undiagnosed with a whole spectrum of medical conditions, including consequential diagnoses of cardiovascular disease, diabetes, and cancer.[370]

"These reported health impacts signal many adults may be having difficulties managing stressors, including grief and trauma, and are likely to lead to significant, long-term individual and societal consequences, including chronic illness and additional strain on the nation's healthcare system."[371]

— American Psychological Association

Key survey findings include:

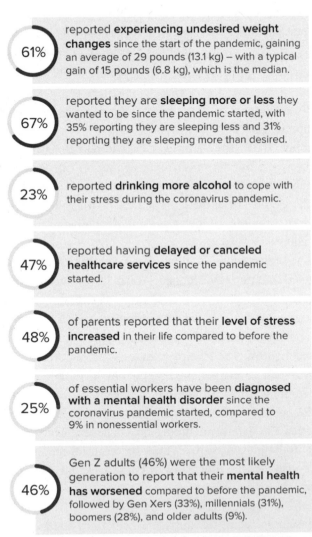

61% reported **experiencing undesired weight changes** since the start of the pandemic, gaining an average of 29 pounds (13.1 kg) — with a typical gain of 15 pounds (6.8 kg), which is the median.

67% reported they are **sleeping more or less** they wanted to be since the pandemic started, with 35% reporting they are sleeping less and 31% reporting they are sleeping more than desired.

23% reported **drinking more alcohol** to cope with their stress during the coronavirus pandemic.

47% reported having **delayed or canceled healthcare services** since the pandemic started.

48% of parents reported that their **level of stress increased** in their life compared to before the pandemic.

25% of essential workers have been **diagnosed with a mental health disorder** since the coronavirus pandemic started, compared to 9% in nonessential workers.

46% Gen Z adults (46%) were the most likely generation to report that their **mental health has worsened** compared to before the pandemic, followed by Gen Xers (33%), millennials (31%), boomers (28%), and older adults (9%).

*Source: American Psychological Association: STRESS IN AMERICA 2021.
One year later, a new wave of pandemic health concerns. March 11, 2021.
https://www.apa.org/news/press/releases/stress/2021/one-year-pandemic-stress*

Developing Resiliency

How we prepare for a traumatic event and avoid its adverse effects is known as resilience. Recall in our last chapter that we talked about perceived control and telomere health. Activating a predictable stress response that is controllable leads to resiliency. To achieve this state, you need to acquire a series of data points and develop healthy habits before the onset of an unexpected stressful or traumatizing event. Like an athlete preparing for their big event, they train. Therefore, you also need to prepare and perform every day to the best of your ability for a significant health event that hopefully will never transpire.

How to Develop Post-Pandemic Health Resiliency

- Acknowledge the impact of the traumatic and recurrent lockdown events.
- Assess the toll the pandemic has caused.
- Repair the damage.
- Recover the body and mind.

And now the final step: reclaiming and renewing our lives post-pandemic. Being proactive is essential, since taking a preventive health strategy could save your life!

Here are your top 10 health action takeaways:

1. **Reduce glycation:** Consuming sugars increases your likelihood of developing metabolic syndrome, leading to diabetes, heart disease, and cancer.
2. **Reduce inflammation:** When tissues are infected or injured, an inflammatory response is created to heal and repair. Scarring can even lead to impaired organ function.
3. **Reduce oxidative stress:** The effect of oxygen and the creation of free radicals can damage your DNA and tissues.
4. **Improve hormonal balance:** Your hormonal "soup" is in constant flux, affecting your metabolic function, especially during physical or emotional stress, pregnancy, and andropause or menopause.

5. **Optimize your nutrient levels:** Food is your first-line drug, and, as such, without the perfect balance of carbohydrates, proteins, and fats, disease can result.

6. **Maintain a steady level of physical fitness:** Exercise and staying active keep all your vascular and lymphatic circulation moving to remove harmful materials and bring in nutrients necessary for growth and repair.

7. **Get enough good quality sleep:** At night, your body recharges, and without good sleep, your hormones go out of sync and this results in impaired metabolism.

8. **Reduce your perceived level of stress:** Take on manageable amounts of physical and emotional challenges in your life. If you feel overwhelmed, ask for help.

9. **Make time to relax:** There are many effective ways to unwind and ease up on the tension you are feeling. Remember to breathe, try yoga, meditate, or engage in other contemplative activities.

10. **Find your life purpose:** It's a surefire way to help re-lengthen your telomeres. Your goal is to live a longer, healthier life, free of chronic diseases, and to be happy and thrive.

Behavioral Change

Habits that served you well before the pandemic may not serve you well now, so you need to let some of them go. Top of mind are all the maladaptive behaviors we discussed in this book, including bad eating habits, lack of impactful exercise, poor sleep habits, and the overuse of alcohol and drugs. We also need to address why you have developed health issues, such as obesity, high blood pressure, and sleep apnea – which negatively impact health outcomes, including COVID-19.

By reading this book, you've already taken a huge step. It has helped to rewire how you think about your health. Your brain is now different because you have acquired new data and assimilated that information into your psyche. We've created new neuro pathways to health. Let's not default to old habits. Find new ways to reward yourself.

Reward System

In *The Power of Habit: Why We Do What We Do in Life and Business,* Pulitzer Prize–winning reporter Charles Duhigg writes that habits consist of a three-step loop:

1. A **cue** triggers your brain to automatically begin your habit or routine.
2. The cue causes you to engage in a physical or mental **routine**, or experience an emotional response.
3. A **reward** or positive reinforcement solidifies the habit.

To change an old habit, replace the undesired routine with a new one, but ensure you get a similar, if not the same, reward. When your brain expects and receives a reward, you are more likely to stick to your new routine.[372]

Finding the motivation to change means we have to make a conscious decision to respond differently to a trigger than we have before. Work done at MIT shows that there is a simple neurological habit loop in our brains.[373]

Here's a simple example. When you are thirsty (which is a physical discomfort cue), your routine is to get something to drink. Once you ingest some water, you are rewarded by your lack of thirst. If, however, the drink is coffee, the reward is complex. On the surface, you've satisfied your thirst, but the caffeine acts as a stimulant. Once the stimulant is metabolized, you may experience a letdown – and now you have two cues, thirst and drug-withdrawal effects, which are harder to resolve. Having too much coffee can result in a habit loop, which can result in a chemical addiction.

This simple and yet potentially complex loop highlights the importance of fully understanding your cues, routines, and rewards. One additional part of this loop is the effect of cravings. Unfortunately, cravings are often chemical in nature. Caffeine is one, and so is sugar. Alcohol, components of tobacco and drugs, and endorphins from (over) exercising are others.

The act of responding habitually to cravings can't be eradicated because the cues in our lives will always be there. Instead, we must replace how we respond to them. Most often, this is our routine response. Once you identify your undesired habit loop, you can begin to find ways to replace your old routines with new ones.

As you experiment to find new routines, also try to change the reward, because rewards have a powerful effect on the cravings response. For example, many of my patients reward themselves with alcohol after a stressful day. As you know, alcohol and telomere health don't mix. Instead, how about having a nice piece of dark chocolate, which has antioxidants? By testing out different rewards, you can determine which craving you are also trying to satisfy or remove.

Motivation

One of the hardest things to do is to change how we behave. According to behavioral scientist Dr. B.J. Fogg of the Persuasive Technology Lab at Stanford University, behavioral change will happen only when three elements converge at the same moment: motivation, ability, and a trigger. When behavioral change does not occur, at least one of those three elements is missing.

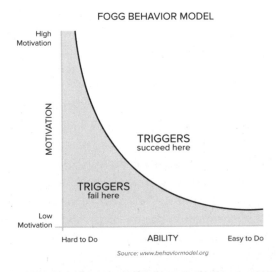

The Fogg Behavior Model has three essential elements that must converge for behavior change: motivation, ability, and a trigger.

SUBCOMPONENTS OF THE 3 FACTORS
FOGG BEHAVIOR MODEL

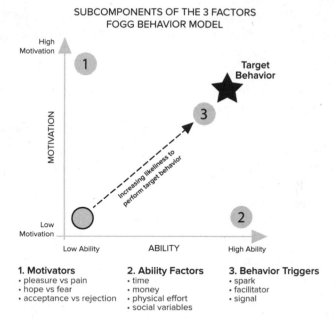

1. Motivators
• pleasure vs pain
• hope vs fear
• acceptance vs rejection

2. Ability Factors
• time
• money
• physical effort
• social variables

3. Behavior Triggers
• spark
• facilitator
• signal

Subcomponents of the three factors in the Fogg Behavior Model.

According to Dr. Fogg, the best time to change habits is when our motivation is high.[374] I can think of no greater motivation than how the microtraumas of this pandemic have impacted our physical and mental well-being. It's time to do something to improve our health resiliency.

Accountability

Remember to gather new data points by performing tests to see how well your mind and body have coped with the COVID-19 pandemic. Numbers don't lie! If the metrics show you are not as well as you'd like to be, this book gave you new approaches and tools to become healthier and more resilient again. Your physical, biochemical, and brain biomarkers can keep you on track and accountable to achieve your desired health outcomes.

In medicine, all diagnostic results can act as potential triggers. How healthcare professionals communicate this data to you into actionable information is critical to triggering your behavioral change. If I gave you a test result number but provided no context or understanding of its implication to you, you would feel no urgency to change; there would be no trigger. And behavioral change is possible only if a person's environment is conducive to that change.

Finding the time, having the money, and committing to improving yourself are critical components of your ability to change. Let me give you a few examples of some environmental situations that make it harder to change. Starting with diet, we know we should cut out all of the "bad" sugars, improve the quality of proteins, and promote a diet full of "good" fats. But if you are spending all your time on road trips and at hockey rinks or baseball diamonds, you may lack the environment to prepare healthy meals – and behavioral change is impossible.

Exercise requires a time commitment of at least several hours a week. Although some people say they need to belong to a gym to work out, I beg to differ. Lots can be done with a skipping rope and a pair of running shoes. If you work 60 hours a week or have very young children or are caring for your aging parents, you may feel you don't have the time to commit to exercise, and this mentality pulls behavioral change out of reach. Take some time for your own health. It's essential.

Achieving an excellent quality of sleep is hard to come by if you do shift work. In fact, this type of sleep cycle practically guarantees bad sleep. Finding a different job may be difficult, but an effort needs to be made to find employment that doesn't harm your health and in an environment that provides for healthy behavioral change.

I recognize that changing habits is hard; routines are ingrained into our day-to-day lives. If we didn't have routines and habits, everything we did would feel like such a challenge because we'd struggle trying to make hundreds, even thousands, of decisions every day. A Duke University study suggests that more than 40% of our actions each day are, in fact, habits.[375]

How do we change or break a habit? With willpower. But this often begs the next question: Am I strong enough? Does it seem like we're asking ourselves to do something strenuous? Well, in fact, we are – because willpower is like a brain muscle. If you haven't used it in a while, it needs retraining. Your willpower is strongest when you believe that you can, in fact, change. To bring about change, you must believe in yourself.

Most often, that belief only emerges with the support of a group. Your odds of success improve dramatically when you commit to changing as part of a group, and change grows out of a communal experience – even if that "group" is only as large as two people.

That is why health professionals are so important to your world. They can function as health coaches, supporting you emotionally. But if your health support is distant and clinical, you might consider finding a health coach who's more engaged with your journey to better health. Lots of healthcare professionals can provide you with medical and factual information. But they're also there to encourage you when you think you can't do what you set out to do.

Until your new, healthier activity becomes a routine or habit, it will be difficult to sustain. Your doctor or health team is there to support you with your challenge of change.

A 2015 study by the American Society of Training and Development found that individuals have the following probabilities of completing a goal by taking these actions. Accountability is key.[376]

- Have an idea or goal: 10% likely to complete the goal.
- Consciously decide that you will do it: 25%.
- Decide when you will do it: 40%.
- Plan how to do it: 50%.
- Commit to someone that you will do it: 65%.
- Have a specific accountability appointment with someone you've committed to: 95%.

But How Do You Practice Accountability?

1. **Ask someone.** You need a compassionate live human who you can trust. A tracking app or a bot is a good start, but you can turn these types of digital support off.
2. **Agree on a plan.** As noted in the research, planning can provide you with a 50% success rate to achieve your goal. This plan needs to include a timeline, action item details, and who may be doing the behavioral change with you.

3. **Take action.** Armed with your plan, it's time to do the work you've committed to follow. Whether it is journaling or taking daily walks or meditating, do it! Perhaps you also want to stop certain habits, like smoking or snacking after dinner.
4. **Track progress.** There is no better motivator than to monitor your progress by measuring the metrics you need to achieve your outcome.
5. **Adjust accordingly.** Share your numbers with your coach. Perhaps the way forward to your goals needs to be modified. You learn and adapt as you go.

"When you want something, all the universe conspires in helping you to achieve it."[377]
— *Paulo Coelho de Souza, Brazilian lyricist and novelist and best known for his novel The Alchemist*

Lifestyle Score

The following scoring scale can help highlight the effects of your overall lifestyle habits. Everyone is unique. We have unique likes and dislikes for different foods, workouts, and ways to spend our free time. It's important to find a lifestyle that works for you.

Diet

0: Eats well, does not skip meals, eats balanced meals, periodically indulges in fast foods
1: Does not skip meals, tends to overeat, eats generally balanced and healthy meals
2: Enjoys a dose of fast foods and junk food but does a reasonably good job of eating balanced meals
3: Eats unbalanced meals, tends to eat out, fast foods are often the norm
4: Skips meals, is a poor eater

Alcohol

0: No alcohol

1: Social drinker: 1 to 2 drinks a week

2: Regular drinker: 1 to 2 drinks most nights

3: Heavy drinker: 1 to 2 drinks at least; 3 or more on weekends and at events

4: Alcoholic: alcohol dependency, admission to overuse or abuse

Sleep

0: Generally good: sleeps 7 to 8 hours of good-quality sleep

1: Generally satisfactory: some nights 6 to 7 hours sleep, most nights 7 to 8 hours sleep

2: Chronically sleep-deprived: sleeps less than 6 to 7 hours

3: Monthly regular episodes of significant sleep deprivation, experiences occasional jet lag of 3 to 5 hours of sleep

4: Sleeping difficulties all the time: quality and quantity of sleep are both poor

Smoking history

0: No

1: Occasional smoking in teenage years, second-hand smoke

2: Social smoker: a few cigarettes a week – not more than half a pack a week

3: Regular smoker: half a pack a week to 1 pack per day (ppd)

4: Heavy smoker: more than 1 ppd

Exercise

0: Active life: exercises 2 to 3 times a week – aerobic and weights

1: Regular activities: plays sports and, occasionally, gym-type activities – running, cycling, and weights

2: No regular sports or aerobic routines: walks only

3: Overexercising: runs serial marathons and participates in iron-man/-woman activities

4: Either completely sedentary or obsessed with exercising more than 2 to 3 hours a day

Score: /20. Generally lower scores indicate positive lifestyle behaviors.

A score of 5 or lower means that the most important aspects of your lifestyle are in good balance.

On the other end of the spectrum, if you scored 3 or higher in any one section, it's time to work to lower it.

Are You Languishing?

Laurie Santos, a Yale University psychology professor, asks two simple questions to determine your state of well-being in one of the most popular classes offered at the university, formally known as Psyc 157: Psychology and the Good Life.

1. Do you wake up ready to start your day, or would you rather go back to sleep?
2. Do you have a sense of purpose, or do you find how you spend much of your day to be meaningless?

She says that you are the expert on your sense of flourishing.[378]

Professor Tyler J. VanderWeele leads Harvard University's Human Flourishing Program. He administers a short survey to assess a person's overall physical, mental, and emotional well-being. There is no cutoff score to say a person is flourishing, but the higher the score, the better. As a benchmark, the average was around 70 before the pandemic, and 65 in June 2020.

Flourishing Measure[379]

Domain 1: Happiness and Life Satisfaction

1. Overall, how satisfied are you with life as a whole these days?

   0 = Not Satisfied at All, 10 = Completely Satisfied

2. In general, how happy or unhappy do you usually feel?

   0 = Extremely Unhappy, 10 = Extremely Happy

Domain 2: Mental and Physical Health

3. In general, how would you rate your physical health?

   0 = Poor, 10 = Excellent

4. How would you rate your overall mental health?

   0 = Poor, 10 = Excellent

Domain 3: Meaning and Purpose

5. Overall, to what extent do you feel the things you do in your life are worthwhile?

   0 = Not at All Worthwhile, 10 = Completely Worthwhile

6. I understand my purpose in life.

   0 = Strongly Disagree, 10 = Strongly Agree

Domain 4: Character and Virtue

7. I always act to promote good in all circumstances, even in difficult and challenging situations.

   0 = Not True of Me, 10 = Completely True of Me

8. I am always able to give up some happiness now for greater happiness later.

   0 = Not True of Me, 10 = Completely True of Me

Domain 5: Close Social Relationships

9. I am content with my friendships and relationships.

   0 = Strongly Disagree, 10 = Strongly Agree

10. My relationships are as satisfying as I would want them to be.

    0 = Strongly Disagree, 10 = Strongly Agree

Domain 6: Financial and Material Stability

11. How often do you worry about being able to meet normal monthly living expenses?

    0 = Worry All of the Time, 10 = Do Not Ever Worry

12. How often do you worry about safety, food, or housing?

    0 = Worry All of the Time, 10 = Do Not Ever Worry

Pathway to Flourishing

To heal from the trauma we've all experienced, we need to rebuild the neural pathways that have caused us to feel fear, sadness, and floundering. New positive pathways can be created by repairing the emotionally damaged ones through meaningful human relationships.

According to Dr. Bruce Perry, social isolation makes you much more physiologically at risk from dying prematurely. Because human beings are social creatures, we are neuro-biologically and physiologically intended to be in relationships with others. When we are in the presence of people who give us physical, emotional, and social signals that we belong, our stress response systems are better regulated. Our reward systems get stimulated, which decreases the probability that we will seek maladaptive ways to reward ourselves through drugs or other things. And, in his view, despite whatever your genetics may be, these positive signals push us toward health, and it prolongs our life. So it's all about relationships; relationships are the agent of change.[380]

As life returns to a new normal, we must again celebrate small and big moments in person. There are so many reasons to get together to welcome a new baby to the family, complete funeral rituals, and recognize the graduates who missed their ceremonies at high school or college. It's time to plan weddings and family vacations.

Here's a checklist of five daily actions to move us all toward flourishing:

1. Remember to savor both the small and big victories.
2. Take time to be in the present and notice all the good things around you.
3. Be thankful for all the positive things that have happened.
4. Pay it forward by performing acts of kindness.
5. Try something new to do outside of your comfort zone.

Returning to Work and Social Interactions

We create relationships in many parts of our lives. It begins with our families. However, we also develop long-lasting friendships at school and at our place of work. For many of us, these institutions were removed from our daily lives by lockdowns. Places of worship and clubs for the arts were also closed. Restaurants and gyms were boarded up. During the pandemic, our social fabric and relationships have been ripped from us. We could not see any extended family members or close friends in person. Video calls were not sufficient for social interactions.

> Everyone needs to return to a place where they can build relationships again for their emotional well-being. Relationships give us opportunities for healing, little iterative moments, all through the day. We get stronger from each other, and we become stronger together.

We are at a critical inflection point of the COVID-19 pandemic. Many employees have continued to suffer from myriad emotional and physical stressors that have left them feeling depressed or burned out.

The 2021 MetLife's 19th Annual U.S. Employee Benefit Trends Study published in March 2021 reports that[381]:

> 37% of employees felt stressed, 22% felt depressed, and 34% felt burned out while working more than half the time, a 7%, 30%, and 25% jump, respectively, compared to April 2020.

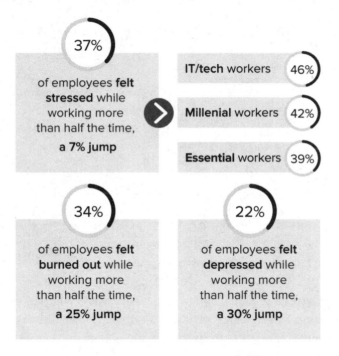

Most strikingly, most employees did not recognize they met the WHO criteria for burnout. Seventy percent of employees said they experienced the following symptoms of burnout since the pandemic began.

Burnout

In May 2019, the WHO defined *burnout* in their *International Classification of Diseases 11th* Revision (ICD-11) as follows: "Burnout is a syndrome conceptualized as resulting from chronic workplace stress that has not been successfully managed."

It is characterized by three dimensions:

1. Feelings of energy depletion or exhaustion
2. Increased mental distance from one's job, or feelings of negativism or cynicism related to one's job
3. Reduced professional efficacy

Burnout "refers specifically to phenomena in the occupational context and should not be applied to describe experiences in other areas of life."[382]

Innovation Health Group published a white paper in May 2021, where I was the lead researcher. Our team found Canadian employees across all industries were anxiously anticipating more meaningful communication and direction from their leadership.

One of the key takeaways was more than 88% of employees said their employers have yet to communicate a coherent COVID-19 vaccination policy to help get them back to the workplace. It's an eye-opening finding that helps to underscore that now more than ever, employees need to know and feel that their employer is providing effective health and safety support before they are willing to return to their workplace.

While those we surveyed continue to have concerns about the safety (41%) and efficacy (44%) of COVID-19 vaccines, the vast majority (84% of employees) have decided to get their vaccines. As a physician, what was most disheartening to me was discovering that health practitioners (20%) were the least sought-out source of information about the vaccines. Yet, we can only assume as a group we are more trusted than traditional and social media.

Our survey also tackled two uncomfortable questions. Should vaccines be mandated to create a higher herd immunity among team members? And can we use digital passports to monitor immunity in the workplace?

We discovered an opening for leaders to explore the mandating of vaccines, while recognizing the legal concerns in certain types of workplaces for presenting such a policy. We found 62% of employees would favor a mandated approach because they would feel safer returning to work.[383]

Many businesses have already invested in screening COVID-19 protocols and must continue to use rapid antigen and PCR (polymerase chain reaction) testing. It also makes sense to leverage the Internet of Things (IoT) and digital technology.

Vaccine passports have generated much debate globally. Instead, I propose narrowing the scope and introducing a workplace immunity passport to support leaders in documenting their workplace vaccination and immunity status.

Our Innovation Health Group survey also found that nearly 90% of respondents were in favor of or interested in considering a digital app to store their vaccination certificate information. They were equally willing to share their vaccination status anonymously with their employer as a means to ensuring workplace safety.

In addition, organizations should consider offering antibody testing to employees. Knowing that their employees' vaccines have effectively mounted a strong immune response with a high antibody count provides peace of mind.

In-Person Interactions

According to the American Psychological Association, more than 50% of employees feel uneasy about adjusting to in-person interaction once the pandemic ends.[384]

Regardless of the various work styles within each organization, it's incumbent on leadership to clearly articulate their present and future expectations and introduce bold policies to help future-proof their organizations.

The time is now for senior leadership teams to step up with forward-thinking actions that will create and maintain the safest possible workplaces for all employees and prioritize mental health resiliency with innovative approaches.

When Do We Go Back to Normal?

In the months following all the on-again, off-again lockdowns, we must work proactively to normalize the fact that COVID-19 will remain part of our lives, not as a memory, but as a virus among us in our day-to-day interactions with one another. However, normalizing does not mean ignoring the necessity to create a safe and secure environment to collaborate and socialize in person again.

Most citizens appreciate the challenging work and decisions made by many public officials. But it's time to have new thought leadership on how we manage a COVID-19 endemic in the years to come. We need different people at the table, with fresh ideas and a new lens on future issues. Robust conversations are necessary as governments grapple with policies to reignite a global economy.

Perhaps a good place to start is to appoint a new set of public health officials who are less biased with the existing data and who can look at the numbers in a new way. A holistic healthcare team – such as nurses, psychologists, and social workers – needs to speak out about community care outreach and mental health programs for at-risk groups. Economists and small business owners must be heard, not just multinational and national companies. Few have highlighted the importance of financial health to maintain physical and mental health. Beyond infectious disease specialists, we should bring in data scientists with artificial intelligence experience to model all types of data sets so that we can make better decisions with more insightful information. And let us not forget the computer programmers. The reality is, we need more of them to support disease reporting and tracking, and to help us improve the logistics of booster vaccination programs in the future.

We need to accept that there will be uncertainty and even chaos in our lives. COVID-19 has forced us to see the fragility within some sectors of our communities. It has also exposed us to many shortcomings in our healthcare system. We must all strive to do better to improve the lives of all humankind. We must make science and technology more practical if we want to democratize access to personalized wellness for everyone.

> The world needs more decentralized, responsive, consumer-centric digital technology. We need to embrace ways to access health diagnostics and quickly act on the results more easily. And at-home self-testing kits, along with virtual health coaching that connects the physical to the virtual care continuum, need to be accessible to all.

It Begins with N=1, You

Embrace integrative wellness into your life. COVID-19 has taught us that every day we are alive, remember that life is not a dress rehearsal. Do not let the SARS-CoV-2 virus define you, but rather shape you into becoming the person you have desired to become.

> *Live every day to its most whole.*
> *Focus on your physical and mental resilience.*
> *Discover ways to live a longer, healthier life.*
> *Fulfill your life purpose.*

Afterword

Addressing the Health of Our Planet

I would be remiss to complete this book without mentioning that the Earth became healthier during the pandemic – especially in the early days of the first lockdown. Around the world, carbon dioxide (CO_2) emissions reduced by 6.4%, due in most part to a sharp decline in transportation both by car and by plane.

- The United States had the highest decline, a 13% decrease in CO_2 emissions.
- The global energy sector was the hardest hit; emissions fell by 48% from the 2019 total.[385]

However, environmentalists felt this drop in CO_2 emissions was disappointing, given the world had come to a forced and dramatic standstill. The United Nations estimates that the world must cut CO_2 emissions by 7.6% per year for the next decade to meet the goals set in the 2015 Paris Agreement.[386]

However, there is no doubt that the emissions will rise once people and products start to move again as the pandemic restrictions fade and consumer demand increases. Therefore, how will we as humankind meet a CO_2-emission reduction of 7.6% when a pandemic could only lower it by 6.4%?

Earth and its people must learn from the pandemic. We were not prepared, not even for PPE needs, let alone having a global pandemic preparedness playbook in place, to reduce the impact of an unknown virus, which quickly turned into the COVID-19 pandemic. It's hard to address the shortfalls once a crisis begins. No government or agency can build up a PPE supply if we don't have any stockpiles and the rest of the world wants to do the same thing. Unfortunately, we have learned it's tough to deal with a pandemic once the pandemic has begun.

Similarly, the global warming crisis had begun well before the pandemic, and many scientists have warned us of its severe impacts on everyone on the planet. Food and water security are just the beginning. The Intergovernmental Panel on Climate Change warns that human health conditions, especially in tropical regions like Africa, will experience an increase in mosquito populations, thus escalating the risk of malaria, dengue, and other insect-borne infections because of a rising temperature.[387]

The challenge with climate change is that we have only one shot to get it right. There is no vaccine cure for global warming. It's hard work. Real work. We must make a more significant and worldwide collective effort to curb emissions, especially when the pandemic has shown us how much more we must do, and in different ways. Acting today to reduce risk tomorrow is essential.

> You are not safe until all of us are safe, including our planet, Earth. We are one.

Acknowledgements

As a family physician with a focus on wellness and personalized medicine, everything I have done over the years to encourage my patients to take more ownership of their healthcare has been reinforced by the global pandemic we have all experienced. So I would be remiss if I did not engage in what I hope is a transformative conversation about how to recover from the biggest health crisis of our generation.

Welcome Back! is a book inspired by you. I've heard from so many people throughout this crisis who now realize just how vital it is to look after ourselves, because without our health we have nothing. Everyone now wants to take better care of themselves and improve their physical and mental resiliency.

In 2015, I wrote my first book, *Lifelines: Unlock the Secrets of Your Telomeres for a Longer, Healthier Life.* The book was inspired by Kenneth Whyte, a distinguished editor of national newspapers and magazines. We made a friendly bet that if he started eating fish, something that is part of a healthy diet, I would take the plunge and write this book. Well, guess, what? Ken started to incorporate fish into his diet, and he held me to the friendly wager.

I must admit, it wasn't easy. Writing has never been my forte, but Ken reminded me that this skill was a muscle too, just like healthy habits. Despite just how challenging the writing process was, I'm very proud of the fact that with a great deal of support and help, my first book became a Top 10 Globe and Mail non-fiction book.

This book has been made possible by Ken again. Here's the back story to how this book came into being. After retiring from his last corporate job, Ken was able to do something he also dreamed of doing, launching his own publishing company, Sutherland House. In late November 2020, I decided to pick up the phone and called him about an idea. I told him to sit down and jokingly said I was sober and not crazy. I told him I've gotten much better at writing and needed to share important advice on how to rebound from the pandemic. He listened to my idea and asked me to send him a book proposal.

Days later, he called me back and said he would publish my book! He agreed with me that it was a timely and important message. Everyone needs to find a new path forward to a healthier life. His only request was to get him the book manuscript in six months.

I was so humbled that one of the best in the business had that kind of faith in me, and of course I told Ken I could do it.

With focused effort and a big lift from Kelly Jones, I delivered the manuscript to Sutherland House in just under seven months. Kelly was on my *Lifelines* team so everything just clicked into place. As impatient as I was to get the writing done, she remained laser focused on her expert editing and fact-checking skills and helped keep me on track to deliver on time. I am grateful to her for her patience and willingness to push back when more work was needed to fine tune the writing and get it right. She knew me well enough to tell me when I needed to do better.

Since my last book, I've met another amazing talent who played a big role in making this book happen. Marie-France Corriveau is a graphics designer who joined my team to help transform ideas into incredible visuals. Check out all our brands and services she helped me launch at www.innovationhealthgroup.com. The graphics in this book are just a sample of her wonderful work and I'm so appreciative of her collaboration on this project.

Welcome Back! has also been motivated by the work I've embarked on with the Four Seasons hotel team in Toronto. Together we are creating a new medispa concept anchored by medical wellness at the Spa at the Four Seasons Toronto. As we began to create wellness offerings, the concepts of repair, recover, and renew became the foundational pillars for this book. Thanks to the entire Four Seasons team for pushing through construction during lockdown to build out our Bespoke Wellness Club space.

As we prepare to put the worst of the pandemic behind us and launch into a new normal, my team at Innovation Health Group are working hard with corporate leadership teams on finding new ways to create a safe return to the workplace, along with innovative wellness experiences, and senior team retreats at the Four Seasons Toronto and other locations in the years to come.

Welcome Back! will truly come to life and be a reality in many workplaces and at wellness destinations.

Thank-you to my team for your unrelenting work to help keep our clients, and Canadians, safe with COVID-19 testing and for helping to create Canada's first *Immunity Passport app* and corporate wellness engagement tool, our *Absolute Wellness Challenge app.*

Our team is also poised to play an instrumental role in democratizing access to science-based virtual wellness offerings with *Health-in-a-Box*, self-test diagnostic kits and at-home facials and skincare solutions with *SkinGenesRx.*

Finally, I want to extend a huge debt of gratitude to my long trusted and loyal team member Cheryl Angeles, who has been by my side my on many journeys we have had over the years at Executive Health Centre. This pandemic sadly took Cheryl's mother. Our team was so grief-stricken by her sudden loss. Millions of people have lost loved ones. I too, was overwhelmed with the prospect of losing my friend Cheryl as she fought, and thankfully beat COVID-19.

While I'm in the business of life and death, I can never get used to the fragility of life. That's why it's so important we celebrate personal successes and life events as they present themselves. As well, we should delight ourselves in the joyful moments and be present to acknowledge them.

On a more personal note, as a mother, I'm so incredibly proud of my son for being part of the graduating class of 2021 at Northwestern University in Industrial Engineering. You've earned this degree Robert, with your hard work and perseverance through so much unexpected adversity. Best of luck as you embark on your career at Ernst and Young, Parthenon.

Elaine

Notes

1 Statista. "Number of coronavirus (COVID-19) cases, recoveries, and deaths worldwide as of June 1, 2021." Statista. Accessed 2021 Jun 1. Available at www.statista.com/statistics/1087466/covid19-cases-recoveries-deaths-worldwidewww.statista.com/statistics/1087466/covid19-cases-recoveries-deaths-worldwide.

2 Winfrey O. "Oprah Winfrey's commencement address." 1997 May 30, Wellesley College. Available at www.wellesley.edu/events/commencement/archives/1997commencement/commencementaddress#:~:text=Turn%20your%20wounds%20into%20wisdom,an%20experience%2C%20just%20an%20experience.

3 Greinacher A, Thiele T, Warkentin TE, Weisser K, et al. "Thrombotic thrombocytopenia after ChAdOx1 nCov-19 vaccination." *N Engl J Med*. 2021 Jun 3. 3; 384 (22): 2092–101.

4 Khoury DS, Cromer D, Reynaldi A, Schlub TE, et al. "Neutralizing antibody levels are highly predictive of immune protection from symptomatic SARS-Cov-2 infection." *Nat Med*. 2021 May 17. doi: 10.1038/s41591-021-01377-8.

5 LeDuc JW, Barry MA. "SARS, the first pandemic of the 21st century." *Emerg Infect Dis*. 2004 Nov; 10 (11): e26. doi: 10.3201/eid1011.040797_02.

6 Guest editors: Balint J, Philpott S, Baker R, Strosberg M. "Chapter 3: The 2003 SARS outbreak in Canada: Legal and ethical lessons about the use of quarantine." *Ethics and Epidemics*. 2006 Nov 9; 9: 43–67. doi: 10.1016/S1479-3709(06)09003-0.

7 Institute of Medicine (US) Forum on Microbial Threats; Knobler S, Mahmoud A, Lemon S, et al., editors. *Learning from SARS: Preparing for the Next Disease Outbreak: Workshop Summary*. Washington (DC): National Academies Press (US); 2004. Available at www.ncbi.nlm.nih.gov/books/NBK92467.

8 Schumaker E. "Timeline: How coronavirus got started." ABC News. 2020 Sept 22. Available at https://abcnews.go.com/Health/timeline-coronavirus-started/story?id=69435165.

9   Canadian Press. "Novel coronavirus in Canada: Here's a timeline of COVID-19 cases across the country." CTV News. 2020 Feb 27. Available at www.ctvnews.ca/canada/novel-coronavirus-in-canada-here-s-a-timeline-of-covid-19-cases-across-the-country-1.4829917.

10 Miller H. "In pictures: China is building two hospitals in less than two weeks to combat virus." CNBC News. 2020 Feb 1. Available at www.cnbc.com/2020/01/31/pictures-china-builds-two-hospitals-in-days-to-combat-coronavirus.html.

11 Boodman E, Branswell H. "First COVID-19 outbreak in a U.S. nursing home raises concerns." Stat News. 2020 Feb 9. Available at www.statnews.com/2020/02/29/new-covid-19-death-raises-concerns-about-virus-spread-in-nursing-homes.

12 Nakazawa E, Hiroyasu I, Akabayashi A. "Chronology of COVID-19 cases on the Diamond Princess Cruise Ship and ethical considerations: A report from Japan." *Disaster Med Public Health Prep*. 2020 Aug; 14 (4): 506–13. doi: 10.1017/dmp.2020.50. Epub 2020 Mar 24.

13 Moriarty LF, Plucinski MM, Marston BJ, et al. "Public health responses to COVID-19 outbreaks on cruise ships — worldwide, February–March 2020." *MMWR Morb Mortal Wkly Rep*. 2020; 69: 347–52. DOI: http://dx.doi.org/10.15585/mmwr.mm6912e3external icon. Available at www.cdc.gov/mmwr/volumes/69/wr/mm6912e3.htm.

14 Martin J. "Trump says those on Grand Princess cruise ship should stay on boat so U.S. coronavirus numbers don't go up." Newsweek. 2020 Mar 6. Available at www.newsweek.com/trump-says-those-grand-princess-cruise-ship-should-stay-boat-so-us-coronavirus-numbers-dont-go-1491038.

15 Patel NV. "Why the CDC botches its coronavirus testing." MIT Technology Review. 2020 Mar 5. Available at www.technologyreview.com/2020/03/05/905484/why-the-cdc-botched-its-coronavirus-testing.

16 Ontario Agency for Health Protection and Promotion (Public Health Ontario). "COVID-19 serosurveillance summary - seroprevalence in Ontario: March 27, 2020, to June 30, 2020." Toronto, ON: Queen's Printer for Ontario; 2020. Available at www.publichealthontario.ca/-/media/documents/ncov/epi/2020/07/covid-19-epi-seroprevalence-in-ontario.pdf?la=en.

17 Al-Qahtani M, AlAli S, AbdulRahman A, Salman Alsayyad A, et al. "The prevalence of asymptomatic and symptomatic COVID-19 in a cohort of quarantined subjects." *Int J Infect Dis*. 2021 Jan; 102: 285–8. doi: 10.1016/j.ijid.2020.10.091. Epub 2020 Nov 3.

18 Elfrink T, Guarino B, Mooney C. "CDC reverses itself and says guidelines it posted on coronavirus airborne transmission were wrong." Washington Post. 2020 Sept 21. Available at www.washingtonpost.com/nation/2020/09/21/cdc-covid-aerosols-airborne-guidelines.

19 Apolone G, Montomoli E, Manenti A, Boeri M, et al. "Unexpected detection

of SARS-CoV-2 antibodies in the prepandemic period in Italy." *Tumori*. 2020 Nov 11: 300891620974755.

20 Deslandes A, Berti V, Tandjaoui-Lambotte Y, Chakib Alloui, et al. "SARS-CoV-2 was already spreading in France in late December 2019." *Int J Antimicrob Agents*. 2020 Jun; 55 (6):106006.

21 U.S. Department of Defense. "Coronavirus: Operation Warp Speed." U.S. Department of Defense. 2020 May 15. Available at www.defense.gov/Explore/Spotlight/Coronavirus/Operation-Warp-Speed/#:~:text=Using%20the%20resources%20of%20the,COVID%2D19%20by%20January%202021.

22 Zhang S. "Why a tiny Colorado county can offer COVID-19 tests to every resident." The Atlantic. 2020 Mar 23. Available at www.theatlantic.com/science/archive/2020/03/coronavirus-tests-everyone-tiny-colorado-county/608590.

23 The National News. "Germany's 'Wuhan' has 15 per cent infection rate and low death toll." 2020 Apr 8. The National News. Available at www.thenationalnews.com/world/germany-s-wuhan-has-15-per-cent-infection-rate-and-low-death-toll-1.1004050.

24 Galloway SE, Paul P, MacCannell DR, Johansson, et al. "Emergence of SARS-CoV-2 B.1.1.7 lineage — United States, December 29, 2020–January 12, 2021." *MMWR Morb Mortal Wkly Rep*. 2021 Jan 22; 70 (3): 95–9. doi: 10.15585/mmwr.mm7003e2.

25 Santos de Oliveira MH, Lippi G, Henry BM. "Sudden rise in COVID-19 case fatality among young and middle-aged adults in the south of Brazil after identification of the novel B.1.1.28.1 (P.1) SARS-CoV-2 strain: Analysis of data from the state of Parana." 2021 Mar 26. *medRxiv* 2021.03.24.21254046

26 Triggle N. "Covid-19 vaccine: First person receives Pfizer jab in UK." BBC News. 2020 Dec 8. Available at www.bbc.com/news/uk-55227325.

27 Statista. "Total number of people who have received a coronavirus (COVID-19) vaccine in the United Kingdom (UK), by dose." Statista. 2021 May 27. Available at www.statista.com/statistics/1194668/uk-covid-19-vaccines-administered.

28 Guarino B, Cha AE, Wood J, Witte G. "The weapon that will end the war: First coronavirus vaccine shots given outside trials in U.S." Washington Post. 2020 Dec 14. Available at www.washingtonpost.com/nation/2020/12/14/first-covid-vaccines-new-york.

29 Centers for Disease Control and Prevention. "Science brief: Emerging SARS-CoV-2 variants." Centers for Disease Control and Prevention. 2021 Jan 28. Available at www.cdc.gov/coronavirus/2019-ncov/science/science-briefs/scientific-brief-emerging-variants.html.

30 Zimonjic P, Kapelos V. "Millions of rapid COVID tests gather dust as some provinces use a fraction of their supply." 2021 Feb 10. CBC News. Available at www.cbc.ca/news/politics/rapid-tests-provinces-use-unused-1.5909702.

31   Phillips K. "'Brutally unforgiving,' COVID-19 outbreak at Barrie, Ont., long-term care home claims 49 lives, infects 214." CTV News. 2021 Jan 27. Available at https://barrie.ctvnews.ca/brutally-unforgiving-covid-19-outbreak-at-barrie-ont-long-term-care-home-claims-49-lives-infects-214-1.5284875.

32   Johns Hopkins University and Medicine. "Daily confirmed new cases (7-day moving average)." Johns Hopkins University and Medicine. Accessed 2021 Jun 1. Available at https://coronavirus.jhu.edu/data/new-cases.

33   Panda S. *The circadian code: Lose Weight, Supercharge Your Energy, and Transform Your Health From Morning To Midnight.* New York: Rodale, an imprint of the Crown Publishing Group, 2018.

34   Almandoz JP, Xie L, Schellinger JN, Mathew MS, et al. "Impact of COVID-19 stay-at-home orders on weight-related behaviors among patients with obesity." *Clinical Obesity.* 2020 Jun 9. doi.org/10.1111/cob.12386.

35   Angus Reid Institute. "Worry, gratitude & boredom: As COVID-19 affects mental, financial health, who fares better; who is worse?" Angus Reid Institute. 2020 Apr 27. Available from http://angusreid.org/covid19-mental-health.

36   Morneau Shepell. "Canadians are feeling unprecedented levels of anxiety, according to Mental Health Index." Morneau Shepell. 2020 Apr 9.

37   Brooks SK, Webster RK, Smith LE, Woodland L, et al. "The psychological impact of quarantine and how to reduce it: Rapid review of the evidence." *Lancet.* 2020 Mar 14; 395 (10227): 912–20. doi: 10.1016/S0140-6736(20)30460-8. Epub 2020 Feb 26.

38   Vigo D, Patten S, Pajer K, Krausz M, et al. "Mental health of communities during the COVID-19 pandemic. *Can J Psychiatry.* 2020 Oct; 65 (10): 681–7. doi: 10.1177/0706743720926676. Epub 2020 May 11.

39   Government of British Columbia. "Statistical reports on deaths in British Columbia." Government of British Columbia. 2021 Apr 29. Available at www2.gov.bc.ca/gov/content/life-events/death/coroners-service/statistical-reports.

40   Cunningham PW. "The health 202: Overdose deaths may have topped 90,000 in 2020." The Washington Post. 2021 Apr 7. Available at www.washingtonpost.com/politics/2021/04/07/health-202-overdose-deaths-may-have-topped-90000-2020.

41   Centers for Disease Control and Prevention. "Binge drinking." Centers for Disease Control and Prevention. 2019 Dec 30. Available at www.cdc.gov/alcohol/fact-sheets/binge-drinking.htm.

42   Canadian Centre on Substance Use and Addiction. "CCSA March Omni | Summary Report. Conducted by Nanos for the Canadian Centre on Substance Use and Addiction. Submission 2020-1621." 2020 April. Available at www.ccsa.ca/sites/default/files/2020-04/CCSA-NANOS-Alcohol-Consumption-During-COVID-19-Report-2020-en.pdf.

43   McKinsey and Company. "Diverse employees are struggling the most during COVID-19—here's how companies can respond." McKinsey and

Company. 2020 Nov 17. Available at www.mckinsey.com/featured-insights/ diversity-and-inclusion/diverse-employees-are-struggling-the-most-during-covid-19-heres-how-companies-can-respond#.

44   https://www.bcg.com/publications/2020/helping-working-parents-ease-the-burden-of-covid-19

45   Centre for Addiction and Mental Health. "COVID-19 pandemic adversely affecting mental health of women and people with children." CAMH. 2020 Oct 14. Available at www.camh.ca/en/camh-news-and-stories/ covid-19-pandemic-adversely-affecting-mental-health-of-women-and-people-with-children.

46   McMaster University's Offord Centre for Child Studies. Sept 2020. https:// assets.documentcloud.org/documents/7203244/OPS-Executive-Report-v6-FINAL.pdf

47   Adams-Prassl A, Boneva T, Golin M, Rauh C. "Inequality in the impact of the coronavirus shock: Evidence from real time surveys." 2020 Apr. IZA discussion paper No. 13183.

48   Centre for Addiction and Mental Health. "COVID-19 pandemic adversely affecting mental health of women and people with children." CAMH. 2020 Oct 14. www.camh.ca/en/camh-news-and-stories/covid-19-pandemic-adversely-affecting-mental-health-of-women-and-people-with-children

49   McKinsey and Company. "Women in the workplace." McKinsey and Company. 2020 Sept 30. Available at www.mckinsey.com/featured-insights/ diversity-and-inclusion/women-in-the-workplace.

50   Offord Centre for Child Studies. "Impact of the Covid-19 pandemic on Ontario families with children: Findings from the initial lockdown." McMaster University. 2020 Sept. Available at https://assets.documentcloud. org/documents/7203244/OPS-Executive-Report-v6-FINAL.pdf.

51   Smith SG, Zhang X, Basile KC, Merrick MT, et al. "National Intimate Partner and Sexual Violence Survey: 2015 Data Brief – Updated Release." National Center for Injury Prevention and Control; Centers for Disease Control and Prevention. 2018 Nov. Available at www.cdc.gov/violenceprevention/pdf/ 2015data-brief508.pdf.

52   Fielding S. "In quarantine with an abuser: Surge in domestic violence reports linked to coronavirus." The Guardian. 2020 Apr 3. Available at www.theguardian.com/us-news/2020/ apr/03/coronavirus-quarantine-abuse-domestic-violence.

53   Pefley A. "Experts see rise in child abuse cases tied to COVID-19." CBS 12 News. 2020 May 22. Available at https://cbs12.com/news/local/ experts-see-rise-in-child-abuse-cases-tied-to-covid-19.

54   Caron F, Plancq M-C, Tourneux P , Gouron R, et al. "Was child abuse under-detected during the COVID-19 lockdown?" *Arch Pediatr*. 2020 Oct; 27 (7): 399–400. doi: 10.1016/j.arcped.2020.07.010. Epub 2020 Aug 6.

55 Fenn K. "Pandemic is creating a new type of homelessness, says outreach worker." CBC News. 2020 Oct 12. Available at www.cbc.ca/radio/thecurrent/the-current-for-oct-12-2020-1.5757769/pandemic-is-creating-a-new-type-of-homelessness-says-outreach-worker-1.5757770.

56 Barrera J, Deer K. "Over 450 Indigenous COVID-19 cases across Canada and 7 deaths, reports Yellowhead Institute." CBC News. 2020 May 12. Available at www.cbc.ca/news/indigenous/yellowhead-institute-coronavirus-report-1.5565954.

57 Centers for Disease Control and Prevention. "Health equity considerations and racial and ethnic minority groups." Centers for Disease Control and Prevention. 2021 Apr 19. Available at www.cdc.gov/coronavirus/2019-ncov/community/health-equity/race-ethnicity.html?CDC_AA_refVal=https%3A%2F%2Fwww.cdc.gov%2Fcoronavirus%2F2019-ncov%2Fneed-extra-precautions%2Fracial-ethnic-minorities.html.

58 Khan KS, Torpiano G, McLellan M, Mahmud S. "The impact of socioeconomic status on 30-day mortality in hospitalized patients with COVID-19 infection." *J Med Virol*. 2021 Feb; 93 (2): 995–1001. doi: 10.1002/jmv.26371. Epub 2020 Aug 13.

59 Office for National Statistics. "Deaths involving COVID-19 by local area and socioeconomic deprivation: Deaths occurring between 1 March and 17 April 2020." Office for National Statistics. 2020 May 1. Available at www.ons.gov.uk/peoplepopulationandcommunity/birthsdeathsandmarriages/deaths/bulletins/deathsinvolvingcovid19bylocalareasanddeprivation/deathsoccurringbetween1marchand17april.

60 Brooks SK, Webster RK, Smith LE, Woodland L, et al. "The psychological impact of quarantine and how to reduce it: Rapid review of the evidence." *Lancet*. 2020 Mar 14. 395 (10227), 912–20.

61 Pfefferbaum B, North CS. "Mental health and the COVID-19 pandemic." *N Engl J Med*. 2020 Aug 6; 383 (6): 510–2. doi: 10.1056/NEJMp2008017. Epub 2020 Apr 13.

62 Van Beusekom M. "Health workers, especially minorities, at high risk for COVID, even with PPE." CIDRAP News. 2020 Aug 3. Available at www.cidrap.umn.edu/news-perspective/2020/08/health-workers-especially-minorities-high-risk-covid-even-ppe.

63 Lee AM, Wong JGWS, McAlonan GM, Cheung V, et al. "Stress and psychological distress among SARS survivors 1 year after the outbreak." *Can J Psychiatry*. 2007 Apr; 52 (4): 233–40. doi: 10.1177/070674370705200405.

64 Mak IWC, Chu CM, Pan PC, Yiu MGC, et al. "Long-term psychiatric morbidities among SARS survivors." *Gen Hosp Psychiatry*. Jul–Aug 2009; 31 (4): 318–26. doi: 10.1016/j.genhosppsych.2009.03.001. Epub 2009 Apr 15.

65 Wu P, Fang Y, Guan Z, Fan B, et al. "The psychological impact of the SARS epidemic on hospital employees in China: Exposure, risk perception, and

altruistic acceptance of risk." *Can J Psychiatry*. 2009 May; 54 (5): 302–11. doi: 10.1177/070674370905400504.

66 Wu PE, Styra R, Gold WL. "Mitigating the psychological effects of COVID-19 on health care workers." *CMAJ*. 2020 Apr 27; 192 (17): E459–60. doi: 10.1503/cmaj.200519. Epub 2020 Apr 15.

67 Goalcast. "Top 20 inspiring Oprah Winfrey quotes that will empower you." Goalcast. 2016 Sept 28. Available at www.goalcast.com/2016/09/28/top-20-inspiring-oprah-winfrey-quotes-that-will-empower-you.

68 https://www.bhf.org.uk/~/media/files/publications/large-print/his14lp_heart-rhythms_0512.pdf

69 Vasan RS, Larson MG, Leip EP, Evans JC, et al. "Impact of high-normal blood pressure on the risk of cardiovascular disease." *N Engl J Med*. 2001 Nov 1; 345 (18): 1291–7. doi: 10.1056/NEJMoa003417.

70 National High Blood Pressure Education Program. "The Seventh Report of the Joint National Committee on Prevention, Detection, Evaluation, and Treatment of High Blood Pressure." Bethesda (MD): National Heart, Lung, and Blood Institute (US); 2004 Aug. Blood Pressure and Cardiovascular Risk. Available at www.ncbi.nlm.nih.gov/books/NBK9634.

71 American Heart Association. "Understanding book pressure readings." American Heart Association. Retrieved 2021 May 31. Available at www.heart.org/en/health-topics/high-blood-pressure/understanding-blood-pressure-readings.

72 Fryar CD, Ostchega Y, Hales CM, Zhang G, et al. "Hypertension prevalence and control among adults: United States, 2015–2016." NCHS data brief, no. 289. Hyattsville, MD: National Center for Health Statistics, 2017.

73 Heart and Stroke Foundation of Canada. "High blood pressure." Retrieved May 31, 2021. Heart and Stroke Foundation of Canada. Available at www.heartandstroke.ca/heart-disease/risk-and-prevention/condition-risk-factors/high-blood-pressure.

74 Robitaille C, Dai S, Waters C, Loukine L, et al. "Diagnosed hypertension in Canada: Incidence, prevalence and associated mortality. *CMAJ*. 2012 Jan 10; 184 (1): E49–56. doi: 10.1503/cmaj.101863. Epub 2011 Nov 21. PMID: 22105752; PMCID: PMC3255225.

75 Thomas SJ, Booth JN 3rd, Dai C, Li X, et al. "Cumulative Incidence of Hypertension by 55 Years of Age in Blacks and Whites: The CARDIA Study." *J Am Heart Assoc*. 2018 Jul 11; 7 (14): e007988. doi: 10.1161/JAHA.117.007988. PMID: 29997132; PMCID: PMC6064834.

76 SPRINT MIND Investigators for the SPRINT Research Group; Williamson JD, Pajewski NM, Auchus AP, Bryan RN, et al. "Effect of intensive vs standard blood pressure control on probable dementia: A randomized clinical trial." *JAMA*. 2019 Feb 12; 321 (6): 553–61. doi: 10.1001/jama.2018.21442.

77 Budson AE. "Can controlling blood pressure later in life reduce risk of dementia?" Harvard Health Publishing. 2020 Jun 29. Available at www.

health.harvard.edu/blog/can-controlling-blood-pressure-later-in-life-re-duce-risk-of-dementia-2020062920498.

78 Appel LJ, Moore TJ, Obarzanek E, Vollmer WM, et al. "A clinical trial of the effects of dietary patterns on blood pressure. DASH Collaborative Research Group." *N Engl J Med*. 1997 Apr 17; 336 (16): 1117–24. doi: 10.1056/NEJM199704173361601.

79 U.S. Food and Drug Administration. "Sodium in your diet." U.S. Food and Drug Administration. 2020 Apr 4. Available at www.fda.gov/food/nutrition-education-resources-materials/sodium-your-diet.

80 U.S. Food and Drug Administration. "Sodium in your diet." U.S. Food and Drug Administration. 2020 Apr 4. Available at www.fda.gov/food/nutrition-education-resources-materials/sodium-your-diet.

81 https://www.heartandstroke.ca/heart-disease/risk-and-prevention/condition-risk-factors/high-blood-pressure

82 Rae L. Quotes Collection. Available at www.leticiarae.com.

83 National Heart, Lung and Blood Institute. "How the lungs work." National Heart, Lung and Blood Institute. 2020 Oct 6. Available at www.nhlbi.nih.gov/health-topics/how-lungs-work#:~:text=serious%20health%20problem.,Breathing%20in,and%20outward%20when%20you%20inhale.

84 Benjafield AV, Ayas NT, Eastwood PR, Heinzer R, et al. "Estimation of the global prevalence and burden of obstructive sleep apnoea: A literature-based analysis." *Lancet Respir Med*. 2019 Aug; 7 (8): 687–98. doi: 10.1016/S2213-2600(19)30198-5. Epub 2019 Jul 9.

85 Teo J. "Early detection of silent hypoxia in COVID-19 pneumonia using smartphone pulse oximetry." *J Med Syst*. 2020 Jun 19; 44 (8): 134. doi: 10.1007/s10916-020-01587-6.

86 Levitan R. "The infection that's silently killing coronavirus patients." The New York Times. 2020 Apr 20. Available at www.nytimes.com/2020/04/20/opinion/sunday/coronavirus-testing-pneumonia.html.

87 Centers for Disease Control and Prevention. "People with certain medical conditions." Centers for Disease Control and Prevention. 2021 May 13. Available at www.cdc.gov/coronavirus/2019-ncov/need-extra-precautions/people-with-medical-conditions.html.

88 Kang Z, Luo S, Gui Y, Zhou H, et al. "Obesity is a potential risk factor contributing to clinical manifestations of COVID-19." *Int J Obes (Lond)*. 2020 Dec; 44 (12): 2479–85. doi: 10.1038/s41366-020-00677-2. Epub 2020 Sep 13.

89 Centers for Disease Control and Prevention. "Insulin resistance and diabetes." Centers for Disease Control and Prevention. 2019 Aug 12. Available at www.cdc.gov/diabetes/basics/insulin-resistance.html.

90 Chernyak BV, Popova EN, Prikhodko AS, Grebenchikov OA, et al. "COVID-19 and oxidative stress." *Biochemistry (Mosc)*. 2020 Dec; 85 (12):1543–53. doi: 10.1134/S0006297920120068.

91 Li M, Dong Y, Wang H, Guo W, et al. "Cardiovascular disease potentially contributes to the progression and poor prognosis of COVID-19." *Nutr Metab Cardiovasc Dis*. 2020 Jun 25; 30 (7): 1061–7. doi: 10.1016/j.numecd.2020.04.013. Epub 2020 Apr 18.

92 Dregan A, Charlton J, Chowienczyk P, Gulliford MC. "Chronic inflammatory disorders and risk of type 2 diabetes mellitus, coronary heart disease, and stroke: A population-based cohort study." *Circulation*. 2014 Sep 2; 130 (10): 837–44. doi: 10.1161/CIRCULATIONAHA.114.009990. Epub 2014 Jun 26.

93 Galiatsatos P, Brodsky R. "What does COVID do to your blood?" Johns Hopkins Medicine. 2020 Nov 18. Available at www.hopkinsmedicine.org/health/conditions-and-diseases/coronavirus/what-does-covid-do-to-your-blood.

94 Stone W. "Clots, strokes and rashes. Is COVID-19 a disease of the blood vessels?" NPR. 2020 Nov 5. Available at www.npr.org/sections/health-shots/2020/11/05/917317541/clots-strokes-and-rashes-is-covid-19-a-disease-of-the-blood-vessels.

95 Friso S, Jacques PF, Wilson PW, Rosenberg IH, et al. "Low circulating vitamin B(6) is associated with elevation of the inflammation marker C-reactive protein independently of plasma homocysteine levels." *Circulation*. 2001 Jun 12; 103 (23): 2788–91. doi: 10.1161/01.cir.103.23.2788.

96 Armstrong M, Palakkamanil M, Loroff N, Slobodan J, et al; Scientific Advisory Group. "COVID-19 Scientific Advisory Group Rapid Evidence Brief." Alberta Health Services. 2021 Jan 7. Available at www.albertahealthservices.ca/assets/info/ppih/if-ppih-covid-19-sag-rapid-review-vitamin-d-treatment-and-prevention-covid-19.pdf.

97 Wei X-B, Wang Z-H, Liao X-L, Guo W-X, et al. "Efficacy of vitamin C in patients with sepsis: An updated meta-analysis." *Eur J Pharmacol*. 2020 Feb 5; 868: 172889. doi: 10.1016/j.ejphar.2019.172889. Epub 2019 Dec 21.

98 Fisher BJ, Seropian IM, Kraskauskas D, Thakkar JN, et al. "Ascorbic acid attenuates lipopolysaccharide-induced acute lung injury." *Crit Care Med*. 2011 Jun; 39 (6): 1454–60. doi: 10.1097/CCM.0b013e3182120cb8.

99 Hoang BX, Shaw G, Fang W, Han B. "Possible application of high-dose vitamin C in the prevention and therapy of coronavirus infection." *J Glob Antimicrob Resist*. 2020 Dec; 23: 256–62. doi: 10.1016/j.jgar.2020.09.025. Epub 2020 Oct 13.

100 National Institutes of Health. "Vitamin C." National Institutes of Health. 2020 Apr 21. Available at www.covid19treatmentguidelines.nih.gov/adjunctive-therapy/vitamin-c.

101 Equils O, Lekaj K, Fattani S, Wu A. "Proposed mechanism for anosmia during COVID-19: The role of local zinc distribution." *Journal of Translational Science*. 2021 Jan. 7 (1). doi:10.15761/JTS.1000397.

102 Morales D, Rutckeviski R, Villalva M, Abreu H, et al. "Isolation and comparison of α- and β-D-glucans from shiitake mushrooms (Lentinula edodes) with different biological activities." *Carbohydr Polym.* 2020 Feb 1; 229: 115521. doi: 10.1016/j.carbpol.2019.115521. Epub 2019 Oct 24.

103 Terakawa N, Matsui Y, Satoi S, Yanagimoto H, et al. "Immunological effect of active hexose correlated compound (AHCC) in healthy volunteers: A double-blind, placebo-controlled trial." *Nutr Cancer.* 2008; 60 (5): 643–51. doi: 10.1080/01635580801993280.

104 Gustavson, Allison M., Danilovich, Margaret K., Lessem, Rachel, Falvey, Jason R. Letters to the Editor: Addressing Rehabilitation Needs During a Pandemic: Solutions to Reduce Burden on Acute and Post-Acute Care Vol 21, Issue 7, P995-997, July 01, 2020. doi:https://doi.org/10.1016/j.jamda.2020.06.007

105 Leproult R, Copinschi G, Buxton O, Van Cauter E. "Sleep loss results in an elevation of cortisol levels the next evening." *Sleep.* 1997 Oct; 20 (10): 865–70.

106 Carpenter S. "That gut feeling." Monitor on Psychology, American Psychological Association. 2012 Sept; (43) 8. Available at www.apa.org/monitor/2012/09/gut-feeling.

107 Baltz JW, Lamanh T Le LT. "Serotonin syndrome versus cannabis toxicity in the emergency department." *Clin Pract Cases Emerg Med.* 2020 Mar 2; 4 (2): 171–3. doi: 10.5811/cpcem.2020.1.45410. eCollection 2020 May.

108 Winkelman JW, Buxton OM, Jensen JE, Benson KL, et al. "Reduced brain GABA in primary insomnia: Preliminary data from 4T proton magnetic resonance spectroscopy (1H-MRS)." *Sleep.* 2008 Nov; 31 (11): 1499–506. doi: 10.1093/sleep/31.11.1499.

109 Byun JI, Shin YY, Chung SE, Shin WC. "Safety and efficacy of gamma-aminobutyric acid from fermented rice germ in patients with insomnia symptoms: A randomized, double-blind trial." *J Clin Neurol.* 2018 Jul; 14 (3): 291–5. doi: 10.3988/jcn.2018.14.3.291. Epub 2018 Apr 27.

110 Pretzsch CM, Freyberg J, Voinescu B, Lythgoe D, et al. "Effects of cannabidiol on brain excitation and inhibition systems; a randomised placebo-controlled single dose trial during magnetic resonance spectroscopy in adults with and without autism spectrum disorder." *Neuropsychopharmacology.* 2019 Jul; 44 (8): 1398–405. doi: 10.1038/s41386-019-0333-8. Epub 2019 Feb 6.

111 Grant A. "There's a name for the blah you're feeling: it's called languishing." The New York Times. 2020 Apr 19. Available at www.nytimes.com/2021/04/19/well/mind/covid-mental-health-languishing.html.

112 Rochat de la Vallée E. *A Study of Qi.* London: Monkey Press, 2016.

113 World Health Organization list of common conditions treatable by Chinese Medicine and Acupuncture. https://www.acupuncture.org.uk/

public-content/public-traditional-acupuncture/4026-who-list-of-conditions.html

114 Helms JM. *Acupuncture Energetics*. Berkeley, CA: Medical Acupuncture Publishers, 1996.

115 Darras J-C, Albarède P, de Vernejoul P. "Nuclear medicine investigation of transmission of acupuncture information." *Acupuncture in Medicine*. 1993 May 1. https://doi.org/10.1136/aim.11.1.22.

116 Joshi S, Mohan V. "Pros & cons of some popular extreme weight-loss diets." *Indian J Med Res*. 2018 Nov; 148 (5): 642–7. doi: 10.4103/ijmr. IJMR_1793_18.

117 Alcock J, Maley CC, Aktipis CA. "Is eating behavior manipulated by the gastrointestinal microbiota? Evolutionary pressures and potential mechanisms." *Bioessays*. 2014 Oct; 36 (10): 940–9. doi: 10.1002/bies.201400071. Epub 2014 Aug 8.

118 Lund-Tonnesen S, Berstad A, Schreiner A, Midvedt T. [Clostridium difficile-associated diarrhea treated with homologous feces]." [Article in Norweigan.] *Tidsskr Nor Laegeforen*. 1998 Mar 10; 118 (7): 1027–30.

119 Williams DR. "Earth Fact Sheet." NASA. 2020 Nov 25. Available at https://nssdc.gsfc.nasa.gov/planetary/factsheet/earthfact.html.

120 Farrell NF, Klatt-Cromwell C, Schneider JS. "Benefits and safety of nasal saline irrigations in a pandemic–washing COVID-19 away." *JAMA Otolaryngol Head Neck Surg*. 2020 Sep 1; 146 (9): 787–8. doi: 10.1001/jamaoto.2020.1622.

121 Yuan SL, Matsutani LA, Pasqual Marques A. "Effectiveness of different styles of massage therapy in fibromyalgia: A systematic review and meta-analysis." *Man Ther*. 2015 Apr; 20 (2): 257–64. doi: 10.1016/j.math.2014.09.003. Epub 2014 Oct 5.

122 Weston M, Taber C, Casagranda L, Cornwall M. "Changes in local blood volume during cold gel pack application to traumatized ankles." *J Orthop Sports Phys Ther*. 1994 Apr; 19 (4): 197–9. doi: 10.2519/jospt.1994.19.4.197.

123 Srámek P, Simecková M, Janský L, Savlíková J, et al. "Human physiological responses to immersion into water of different temperatures." *Eur J Appl Physiol*. 2000 Mar; 81 (5): 436–42. doi: 10.1007/s004210050065.

124 Huttunen P, Kokko L, Ylijukuri V. "Winter swimming improves general well-being." *Int J Circumpolar Health*. 2004 May; 63 (2): 140–4. doi: 10.3402/ijch.v63i2.17700.

125 Mooventhan A, Nivethitha L. "Scientific evidence-based effects of hydrotherapy on various systems of the body." *N Am J Med Sci*. 2014 May; 6 (5): 199–209. doi: 10.4103/1947-2714.132935.

126 Laukkanen T, Khan H, Zaccardi F, Laukkanen JA. "Association between sauna bathing and fatal cardiovascular and all-cause mortality events." *JAMA Intern Med*. 2015 Apr; 175 (4): 542–8. doi: 10.1001/jamainternmed.2014.8187.

127 Laukkanen T, Kunutsor S, Kauhanen J, Laukkanen JA. "Sauna bathing is inversely associated with dementia and Alzheimer's disease in middle-aged Finnish men." *Age Ageing*. 2017 Mar 1; 46 (2): 245–9. doi: 10.1093/ageing/afw212.

128 Hannuksela ML, Ellahham S. "Benefits and risks of sauna bathing." *Am J Med*. 2001 Feb 1; 110 (2): 118–26. doi: 10.1016/s0002-9343(00)00671-9.

129 Russ TC, Stamatakis E, Hamer M, Starr JM, et al. "Association between psychological distress and mortality: Individual participant pooled analysis of 10 prospective cohort studies." *BMJ*. 2012 Jul 31; 345: e4933. doi: 10.1136/bmj.e4933.

130 Chiba S, Numakawa T, Ninomiya M, Richards MC, et al. "Chronic restraint stress causes anxiety- and depression-like behaviors, downregulates glucocorticoid receptor expression, and attenuates glutamate release induced by brain-derived neurotrophic factor in the prefrontal cortex." *Prog Neuropsychopharmacol Biol Psychiatry*. 2012 Oct 1; 39 (1): 112–9. doi: 10.1016/j.pnpbp.2012.05.018. Epub 2012 Jun 1.

131 MetLife. "Redesigning the employee experience: Preparing the workforce for a transformed world," MetLife's 19th Annual U.S. Employee Benefit Trends Study 2021. Available at www.metlife.com/ebts2021.

132 Uchakin PN, Tobin B, Cubbage M, Marshall G Jr, et al. "Immune responsiveness following academic stress in first-year medical students." *J Interferon Cytokine Res*. 2001 Sep; 21 (9): 687–94. doi: 10.1089/107999001753124426. PMID: 11576463.

133 American Psychology Association. "Stress weakens the immune system." American Psychology Association. 2006 Feb 23. Available at www.apa.org/research/action/immune.

134 Field T, Hernandez-Reif M, Diego M, Schanberg S, et al. "Cortisol decreases and serotonin and dopamine increase following massage therapy." *Int J Neurosci*. 2005 Oct; 115 (10): 1397–413. doi: 10.1080/00207450590956459.

135 Heppner WL, Kernis MH. "'Quiet ego' functioning: The complementary roles of mindfulness, authenticity, and secure high self-esteem." *Psychological Inquiry*. 2007 Oct. 18 (4), 248–51. https://doi.org/10.1080/10478400701598330.

136 Weinstein N, Brown KW, Ryan RM. "A multi-method examination of the effects of mindfulness on stress attribution, coping and, emotional well-being." *J Res in Pers*. 2009; 43: 374–85. doi: 10.1016/j.jrp.2008.12.008.

137 Epel E, Daubenmier J, Moskowitz JT, Folkman S, et al. "Can meditation slow rate of cellular aging? Cognitive stress, mindfulness, and telomeres." *Ann N Y Acad Sci*. 2009 Aug; 1172: 34–53. doi: 10.1111/j.1749-6632.2009.04414.x.

138 Dallman MF, Akana SF, Strack AM, Hanson ES, et al. "The neural network that regulates energy balance is responsive to glucocorticoids and insulin and also regulates HPA axis responsivity at a site proximal to CRF neurons." *Ann N Y Acad Sci*. 1995 Dec 29; 771: 730–42.

139 McEwen BS. "Protective and damaging effects of stress mediators." *N Engl J Med*. 1998 Jan 15; 338 (3): 171–9. doi: 10.1056/NEJM199801153380307.

140 Adam EK, Gunnar MR. "Relationship functioning and home and work demands predict individual differences in diurnal cortisol patterns in women." *Psychoneuroendocrinology*. 2001 Feb; 26 (2): 189–208. doi: 10.1016/s0306-4530(00)00045-7.

141 Epel E, Burke H, Wolkowitz O. "Psychoneuroendocrinology of aging: Focus on anabolic and catabolic hormones." In: Aldwin C, Spiro A, Park C, editors. *Handbook of Health Psychology of Aging*. New York: Guildford Press; 2007. pp. 119–41.

142 MetLife. "Redesigning the employee experience: Preparing the workforce for a transformed world," MetLife's 19th Annual U.S. Employee Benefit Trends Study 2021. Available at www.metlife.com/ebts2021.

143 Hall DE. "Religious attendance: More cost-effective than Lipitor?" *J Am Board Fam Med*. 2006 Mar–Apr; 19 (2): 103–9. doi: 10.3122/jabfm.19.2.103.

144 Schnall E, Wassertheil-Smoller S, Swencionis C, Zemon V, et al. "The relationship between religion and cardiovascular outcomes and all-cause mortality in the women's health initiative observational study." *Psychol Health*. 2010 Feb; 25 (2): 249–63. doi: 10.1080/08870440802311322.

145 Bower JE, Low CA, Moskowitz JT, Sepah S, et al. "Benefit finding and physical health: Positive psychological changes and enhanced allostasis." *Social and Personality Psychology Compass*. 2008; 2 (1): 223–44.

146 Washington State University. "Stress reduction benefits from petting dogs, cats." *Science Daily*. 2019 Jul 15. Available at www.sciencedaily.com/releases/2019/07/190715114302.htm.

147 Olsen C, Pedersen I, Bergland A, Enders-Slegers MJ, et al. "Effect of animal-assisted interventions on depression, agitation and quality of life in nursing home residents suffering from cognitive impairment or dementia: A cluster randomized controlled trial." *Int J Geriatr Psychiatry*. 2016 Dec; 31 (12): 1312–21.

148 O'Haire ME, Guérin NA, Kirkham AC. "Animal-assisted intervention for trauma: A systematic literature review." *Front Psychol*. 2015 Aug 7; 6: 1121. doi:10.3389/fpsyg.2015.01121.

149 Pendry P, Carr AM, Roeter SM, Vandagriff JL. "Experimental trial demonstrates effects of animal-assisted stress prevention program on college students' positive and negative emotion." *Human-Animal Interaction Bulletin*. 2018. 6 (1), 81–97.

150 Barker SB, Barker RT, McCain NL, et al. "A randomized cross-over exploratory study of the effect of visiting therapy dogs on college student stress before final exams." *Anthrozoos A Multidisciplinary Journal of the Interactions of People & Animals*. 2016 Jan. 29 (1), 35–46. doi:10.1080/0 8927936.2015.1069988.

151 Grajfoner D, Harte E, Potter, LM, McGuigan N. "The effect of a dog-assisted intervention on student well-being, mood, and anxiety." *Int. J. Environ. Res. Public Health.* 2017 May 5. 14 (5), 483; https://doi.org/10.3390/ijerph14050483.

152 Pendry P, Vandagriff JL. "Animal visitation program (AVP) reduces cortisol levels of university students: A randomized controlled trial." *AERA Open.* 2019 June 12. doi: 10.1177/2332858419852592.

153 Martin L, Oepen R, Bauer K, Nottensteiner A, et al. "Creative arts interventions for stress management and prevention—a systematic review." *Behav Sci (Basel).* 2018 Feb; 8 (2): 28. doi: 10.3390/bs8020028.

154 PabloPicasso.Org. "Pablo Picasso's Blue Period – 1901 to 1904." Available at www.pablopicasso.org/blue-period.jsp.

155 Oepen R, Gruber H. [An art therapy project day to promote health for clients from burnout self-help groups--an exploratory study]. *Psychother Psychosom Med Psychol.* 2014 Jul; 64 (7): 268–74. German. doi: 10.1055/s-0033-1358725. Epub 2013 Dec 16. PMID: 24343313.

156 Herrmann N. "What is the function of the various brainwaves?" *Scientific American.* 1997 Dec 22. Available at www.scientificamerican.com/article/what-is-the-function-of-t-1997-12-22.

157 Saarman E. "Feeling the beat: Symposium explores the therapeutic effects of rhythmic music." 2006 May 31. *Stanford News.* Available at https://news.stanford.edu/news/2006/may31/brainwave-053106.html.

158 Acolin J. "The mind–body connection in dance/movement therapy: Theory and empirical support." *Am J Dance Ther.* 2016 Aug 26. 38, 311–33. https://doi.org/10.1007/s10465-016-9222-4.

159 Strauss J. "Sour mood getting you down? Get back to nature: Research suggests that mood disorders can be lifted by spending more time outdoors." *Harvard Men's Health Watch.* Jul 2018. 22 (12): 3.

160 Meredith GR, Rakow DA, Eldermire ERB, Madsen CG, et al. "Minimum time dose in nature to positively impact the mental health of college-aged students, and how to measure it: A scoping review." *Front Psychol.* 2020 Jan 14; 10: 2942. doi: 10.3389/fpsyg.2019.02942. eCollection 2019.

161 National Academies of Sciences, Engineering, and Medicine; Health and Medicine Division; Board on Population Health and Public Health Practice; Committee on the Health Effects of Marijuana. *An Evidence Review and Research Agenda. The Health Effects of Cannabis and Cannabinoids: The Current State of Evidence and Recommendations for Research.* Washington (DC): National Academies Press (US); 2017 Jan 12. 4

162 Verbeke R, Lentacker I, De Smedt SC, Dewitte H. "Three decades of messenger RNA vaccine development." *Nano Today.* 2019 Oct. 28: 100766.

163 Dolgin E. "Unlocking the potential of vaccines built on messenger RNA."

Nature. 2019 Oct; 574 (7778): S10–2. doi: 10.1038/d41586-019-03072-8. PMID: 31619807.

164 Taylor P. "Regeneron pairs with BioNTech on melanoma immunotherapy." *PharmaPhorum.* 2020 Aug 3. Available at https://pharmaphorum.com/news/regeneron-pairs-with-biontech-on-melanoma-immunotherapy.

165 Bray GA. "The epidemic of obesity and changes in food intake: the fluoride hypothesis." *Physiol Behav.* 2004 Aug; 82 (1): 115–21. doi: 10.1016/j.physbeh. 2004.04.033.

166 Jackson SE, Llewellyn CH, Smith L. "The obesity epidemic – nature via nurture: A narrative review of high-income countries." *SAGE Open Med.* 2020 Apr 28; 8: 2050312120918265. doi: 10.1177/2050312120918265. eCollection 2020.

167 Llewellyn, CH, Fildes, A. "Behavioural susceptibility theory: Professor Jane Wardle and the role of appetite in genetic risk of obesity." *Curr Obes Rep.* 2017 Mar; 6 (1): 38–45. doi: 10.1007/s13679-017-0247-x.

168 Centers for Disease Control and Prevention. "Trends in intake of energy and macronutrients—United States, 1971–2000." Centers for Disease Control and Prevention. 2004 Feb 6. Available at www.cdc.gov/mmwr/preview/mmwrhtml/mm5304a3.htm.

169 Stoll LL, McCormick ML, Denning GM, Weintraub NL. "Antioxidant effects of statins." *Drugs Today (Barc).* 2004 Dec; 40 (12): 975–90. doi: 10.1358/dot.2004.40.12.872573.

170 Chow R. "The protective association between statins use and adverse outcomes among COVID-19 patients: A systematic review and meta-analysis." *MedRxiv.* 2021 Feb 9. Available at www.medrxiv.org/content/10.1101/2021.02.08.21251070v1.

171 Lustig RH. "Sugar: The Bitter Truth" YouTube video. University of California Television. 2009 Jul 30. Available at htwww.youtube.com/watch?v=dBnniua6-oM.

172 Sclafani A, Springer D. "Dietary obesity in adult rats: Similarities to hypothalamic and human obesity syndromes." *Physiol Behav.* 1976 Sep; 17 (3): 461–71. doi: 10.1016/0031-9384(76)90109-8.

173 Moss M. *Salt Sugar Fat: How the Food Giants Hooked Us.* New York: Random House, 2013.

174 Stanhope KL, Bremer AA, Medici V, Nakajima K, et al. "Consumption of fructose and high fructose corn syrup increase postprandial triglycerides, LDL-cholesterol, and apolipoprotein-B in young men and women." *J Clin Endocrinol Metab.* 2011 Oct; 96 (10): E1596–605. doi: 10.1210/jc.2011-1251.

175 Mathur K, Agrawal RK, Nagpure S, Deshpande D. "Effect of artificial sweeteners on insulin resistance among type-2 diabetes mellitus patients." *J Family Med Prim Care.* 2020 Jan 28; 9 (1): 69–71. doi: 10.4103/jfmpc.jfmpc_329_19.

176   Fowler SP, Williams K, Resendez RG, Hunt KJ, et al. "Fueling the obe-
      sity epidemic? Artificially sweetened beverage use and long-term weight
      gain." *Obesity (Silver Spring)*. 2008 Aug; 16 (8): 1894–900. doi: 10.1038/
      oby.2008.284. Epub 2008 Jun 5.

177   Swithers SE. "Artificial sweeteners produce the counterintuitive effect of
      inducing metabolic derangements." *Trends Endocrinol Metab*. 2013; 24 (9):
      431–41. doi:10.1016/j.tem.2013.05.005.

178   Thompson M, Hein N, Hanson C, Smith LM, et al. "Omega-3 fatty acid
      intake by age, gender, and pregnancy status in the United States: National
      Health and Nutrition Examination Survey 2003–2014." *Nutrients*. 2019
      Jan 15; 11 (1): 177. doi: 10.3390/nu11010177.

179   Smith KJ, Sanderson K, McNaughton SA, Gall SL, et al. "Longitudinal
      associations between fish consumption and depression in young adults."
      Am J Epidemiol. 2014 May 15; 179 (10): 1228–35. doi: 10.1093/aje/
      kwu050. Epub 2014 Apr 15.

180   Oliver JM, Anzalone AJ, Turner SM. "Protection before impact: the poten-
      tial neuroprotective role of nutritional supplementation in sports-related
      head trauma." *Sports Med*. 2018 Mar; 48 (Suppl 1): 39–52. doi: 10.1007/
      s40279-017-0847-3.

181   Harel Z, Gascon G, Riggs S, Vaz R, et al. "Supplementation with omega-3
      polyunsaturated fatty acids in the management of recurrent migraines in
      adolescents." *J Adolesc Health*. 2002 Aug; 31 (2): 154–61.

182   Appel LJ, Baker DH, Bar-Or O, Minaker KL, et al. "Report sets dietary intake
      levels for water, salt, and potassium to maintain health and reduce chronic
      disease risk." 2004 Feb 11. *National Academies of Sciences, Engineering,
      Medicine*. Available at www.nationalacademies.org/news/2004/02/
      report-sets-dietary-intake-levels-for-water-salt-and-potassium-to-main-
      tain-health-and-reduce-chronic-disease-risk.

183   Mayo Clinic Staff. "Nutrition and healthy eating." Mayo Clinic. 2020 Oct 14.
      Available at www.mayoclinic.org/healthy-lifestyle/nutrition-and-healthy-
      eating/in-depth/water/art-20044256.

184   Mann T, Tomiyama AJ, Westling E, Lew AM, et al. "Medicare's search for
      effective obesity treatments: Diets are not the answer." *Am Psychol*. 2007
      Apr; 62 (3): 220–33.

185   Kim KR, Nam SY, Song YD, Lim SK, et al. "Low-dose growth hormone treat-
      ment with diet restriction accelerates body fat loss, exerts anabolic effect,
      and improves growth hormone secretory dysfunction in obese adults."
      Horm Res. 1999; 51 (2): 78–84. doi: 10.1159/000023319.

186   Walford RL, Weber L, Panov S. "Caloric restriction and aging as viewed
      from Biosphere 2. Receptor." *Receptor*. Spring 1995; 5 (1): 29–33.

187   Fakhrzadeh H, Larijani B, Sanjari M, Baradar-Jalili R, et al. "Effect of
      Ramadan fasting on clinical and biochemical parameters in healthy

adults." *Ann Saudi Med.* May–Jul 2003; 23 (3–4): 223–6. doi: 10.5144/0256-4947.2003.223.

188 National Institutes of Health. "Calorie restriction and fasting diets: What do we know?" National Institutes of Health. 2018 Aug 14. Available at www.nia.nih.gov/health/calorie-restriction-and-fasting-diets-what-do-we-know.

189 Panda S. *The Circadian Code: Lose Weight, Supercharge Your Energy, and Transform Your Health from Morning to Midnight.* New York: Rodale Books, 2020.

190 Przulj D, Ladmore D, Myers Smith K, Phillips-Waller A, et al. "Time-restricted eating as a weight loss intervention in adults with obesity." *PLoS One.* 2021 Jan 28; 16 (1): e0246186. doi: 10.1371/journal.pone.0246186. eCollection 2021.

191 Jakubowicz D, Barnea M, Wainstein J, Froy O. "High-caloric intake at breakfast vs. dinner differentially influences weight loss of overweight and obese women." *Obesity (Silver Spring).* 2013 Dec; 21 (12): 2504–12. doi: 10.1002/oby.20460. Epub 2013 Jul 2.

192 Davis A. "'Eat breakfast like a king, lunch like a prince and dinner like a pauper' in 1955." *Kingsport News.* 1955 Sep 2. Available at www.newspapers.com/clip/33788065/eat-breakfast-like-a-king-lunch-like.

193 Robillard R, Saad M, Edwards J, Solomonova E, et al. "Social, financial and psychological stress during an emerging pandemic: Observations from a population survey in the acute phase of COVID-19." *BMJ Open.* 2020 Dec 12; 10 (12): e043805. doi: 10.1136/bmjopen-2020-043805. PMID: 33310814; PMCID: PMC7735085.

194 Nielsen T. "The COVID-19 pandemic is changing our dreams." *Scientific American.* 2020 Oct. 323, 4, 30–4. Available at www.scientificamerican.com/article/the-covid-19-pandemic-is-changing-our-dreams.

195 Falkingham J, Evandrou M, Qin M, Vlachantoni A. "'Sleepless in lockdown': Unpacking differences in sleep loss during the coronavirus pandemic in the UK." 2020 Jul 21. MedRxiv. Available at www.medrxiv.org/content/10.1101/2020.07.19.20157255v1.

196 Lin L-Y, Wang J, Ou-Yang X-Y, Miao Q, et al. "The immediate impact of the 2019 novel coronavirus (COVID-19) outbreak on subjective sleep status." *Sleep Med.* 2021 Jan; 77: 348–54. doi: 10.1016/j.sleep.2020.05.018. Epub 2020 Jun 1.

197 Voitsidis P, Gliatas I, Bairachtari V, Papadopoulou K, et al. "Insomnia during the COVID-19 pandemic in a Greek population." *Psychiatry Res.* 2020 Jul; 289: 113076. doi: 10.1016/j.psychres.2020.113076. Epub 2020 May 12.

198 Gupta R, Pandi-Perumal SR. "COVID-Somnia: How the pandemic affects sleep/wake regulation and how to deal with it." *Sleep Vigil.* 2020 Dec 3; 1–3. doi: 10.1007/s41782-020-00118-0.

199 Ellis JG, Perlis ML, Neale LF, Espie CA, et al. "The natural history of

insomnia: Focus on prevalence and incidence of acute insomnia." *J Psychiatr Res*. 2012 Oct; 46 (10): 1278–85. doi: 10.1016/j.jpsychires.2012.07.001.

200 Ji X, Ivers H, Savard J, LeBlanc M, et al. "Residual symptoms after natural remission of insomnia: Associations with relapse over 4 years." *Sleep*. 2019 Aug 1; 42 (8): zsz122. doi: 10.1093/sleep/zsz122.

201 Watson N, Badr MS, Belenky G, Bliwise DL, et al. "Joint consensus statement of the American Academy of sleep medicine and sleep research society on the recommended amount of sleep for a healthy adult: Methodology and discussion." *Sleep*. 2015 Aug 1; 38 (8): 1161–83. doi: 10.5665/sleep.4886.

202 Suni E. "Teens and sleep." Sleep Foundation. 2020 Aug 5. Available at www.sleepfoundation.org/teens-and-sleep.

203 Kansagra S. "How America sleeps." Mattress Firm. 2019 May. Available at http://newsroom.mattressfirm.com/wp-content/uploads/2019/05/Better-Sleep-Month-Sleep-Trend-Report.pdf?x91843.

204 Carskadon MA, Harvey K, Duke P, Anders TF, et al. "Pubertal changes in daytime sleepiness." *Sleep*. 2002 Sep 15; 25 (6): 453–60.

205 Chapman DP, Wheaton AG, Perry GS, Sturgis SL, et al. "Household demographics and perceived insufficient sleep among US adults." *J Community Health*. 2012 Apr; 37 (2): 344–9. doi: 10.1007/s10900-011-9451-x.

206 Wickwire EM, Shaya FT, Scharf SM. "Health economics of insomnia treatments: The return on investment for a good night's sleep." *Sleep Med Rev*. 2016 Dec; 30: 72–82. doi: 10.1016/j.smrv.2015.11.004.

207 Olfson M, Wall M, Liu SM, Morin CM, et al. "Insomnia and impaired quality of life in the United States." *J Clin Psychiatry*. 2018 Sep 11; 79 (5): 17m12020. doi: 10.4088/JCP.17m12020.

208 Hafner M, Stepanek M, Taylor J, Troxel WM et al. "Why sleep matters—the economic costs of insufficient sleep: A comparative cross-country analysis." *Rand Health Q*. 2017 Jan 1; 6 (4): 11. eCollection 2017 Jan.

209 NIH: Sleep Deprivation and Deficiency https://www.nhlbi.nih.gov/health-topics/sleep-deprivation-and-deficiency

210 Chattu VK, Sakhamuri SM, Kumar R, Spence DW, et al. "Insufficient sleep syndrome: Is it time to classify it as a major noncommunicable disease?" *Sleep Sci*. Mar–Apr 2018; 11 (2): 56–64. doi: 10.5935/1984-0063.20180013.

211 Chapman DP, Croft JB, Liu Y, Perry GS, et al. "Excess frequent insufficient sleep in American Indians/Alaska natives." *J Environ Public Health*. 2013; 259645. doi: 10.1155/2013/259645. Epub 2013 Feb 21.

212 Hublin C, Kaprio J, Partinen M, Koskenvuo M. "Insufficient sleep—A population-based study in adults." *Sleep*. 2001 Jun 15; 24 (4): 392–400. doi: 10.1093/sleep/24.4.392.

213 Walsh JK, Coulouvrat C, Hajak G, Lakoma MD, et al. "Nighttime insomnia symptoms and perceived health in the America Insomnia Survey (AIS)." *Sleep*. 2011 Aug 1; 34 (8): 997–1011. doi: 10.5665/SLEEP.1150.

214 Kessler RC, Berglund PA, Coulouvrat C, Hajak G, et al. "Insomnia and the performance of U.S. workers: Results from the America insomnia survey." *Sleep*. 2011 Sep 1; 34 (9): 1161–71. doi: 10.5665/SLEEP.1230.

215 Grewal RG, Doghramji K. "Epidemiology of insomnia." In: *Clinical Handbook of Insomnia*. 3rd ed. Attarian HP. Humana Press, ed. 2016

216 Chaput JP, Yau J, Rao DP, Morin CM. "Prevalence of insomnia for Canadians aged 6 to 79." *Health Rep*. 2018 Dec 19; 29 (12): 16–20.

217 Ohayon MM. "Epidemiology of insomnia: What we know and what we still need to learn." *Sleep Med Rev*. 2002 Apr; 6 (2): 97–111. doi: 10.1053/smrv.2002.0186.

218 Bastien CH, Vallieres A, Morin CM. "Precipitating factors of insomnia." *Behav Sleep Med*. 2004; 2 (1): 50–62. doi: 10.1207/s15402010bsm0201_5.

219 Fuller PM, Gooley JJ, Saper CB. "Neurobiology of the sleep-wake cycle: Sleep architecture, circadian regulation, and regulatory feedback." *J Biol Rhythms*. 2006 Dec; 21 (6): 482–93. doi: 10.1177/0748730406294627.

220 Institute of Medicine (US) Committee on Sleep Medicine and Research; Colten HR, Altevogt BM, editors. *Sleep Disorders and Sleep Deprivation: An Unmet Public Health Problem*. Washington (DC): National Academies Press (US); 2006. Available at www.ncbi.nlm.nih.gov/books/NBK19960/ doi: 10.17226/11617.

221 Patel AK, Reddy V, Araujo JF. *Physiology, Sleep Stages*. [Updated 2021 Apr 22]. In: StatPearls [Internet]. Treasure Island (FL): StatPearls Publishing; 2021 Jan-. Available at www.ncbi.nlm.nih.gov/books/NBK526132.

222 Dinges DF, Douglas SD, Hamarman S, Zaugg L, et al. "Sleep deprivation and human immune function." *Adv Neuroimmunol*. 1995; 5 (2): 97–110. doi: 10.1016/0960-5428(95)00002-j.

223 Aho V, Ollila HM, Kronholm E, Bondia-Pons I, et al. "Prolonged sleep restriction induces changes in pathways involved in cholesterol metabolism and inflammatory responses." *Sci Rep*. 2016 Apr 22; 6: 24828. doi: 10.1038/srep24828.

224 Taheri S, Lin L, Austin D, Young T, et al. "Short sleep duration is associated with reduced leptin, elevated ghrelin, and increased body mass index." *PLoS Med*. 2004 Dec; 1 (3): e62. doi: 10.1371/journal.pmed.0010062. Epub 2004 Dec 7.

225 Chatto VK, Manzar MD, Kumar S, Burman D, et al. "The global problem of insufficient sleep and its serious public health implications." *Healthcare (Basel)*. 2018 Dec 20; 7 (1): 1. doi: 10.3390/healthcare7010001.

226 Savage LC. "Go to bed tonight. On time. (Or else.)" *Maclean's*. 2013 Jun 17. Available at www.macleans.ca/society/life/the-sleep-crisis.

227 Knutson KL, Spiegel K, Penev P, Van Cauter E. The metabolic consequences of sleep deprivation. *Sleep Med Rev*. 2007 Jun; 11 (3): 163–78. doi: 10.1016/j.smrv.2007.01.002.

228 Dutil C, Chaput J-P. "Inadequate sleep as a contributor to type 2 diabetes in children and adolescents." *Nutr Diabetes*. 2017 May 8; 7 (5): e266. doi: 10.1038/nutd.2017.19.
229 Penev PD. "Update on energy homeostasis and insufficient sleep." *J Clin Endocrinol Metab*. 2012 Jun; 97 (6): 1792–801. doi: 10.1210/jc.2012-1067.
230 Irwin M, McClintick J, Costlow C, Fortner M, et al. "Partial night sleep deprivation reduces natural killer and cellular immune responses in humans." *FASEB J*. 1996 Apr; 10 (5): 643–53. doi: 10.1096/fasebj.10.5.8621064.
231 Prather AA, Leung CW. "Association of insufficient sleep with respiratory infection among adults in the United States." *JAMA Intern Med*. 2016 Jun 1; 176 (6): 850–2. doi: 10.1001/jamainternmed.2016.0787.
232 Markt SC, Grotta A, Nyren O, Adami HO, et al. "Insufficient sleep and risk of prostate cancer in a large Swedish cohort." *Sleep*. 2015 Sep 1; 38 (9): 1405–10. doi: 10.5665/sleep.4978.
233 Lehrer S, Green S, Ramanathan L, Rosenzweig KE. "Insufficient sleep associated with increased breast cancer mortality." *Sleep Med*. 2013 May; 14 (5): 469. doi: 10.1016/j.sleep.2012.10.012. Epub 2013 Mar 6.
234 Chattu VK, Manzar MD, Kumary S, Burman D, et al. "The global problem of insufficient sleep and its serious public health implications." *Healthcare (Basel)*. 2018 Dec 20; 7 (1): 1. doi: 10.3390/healthcare7010001. PMID: 30577441; PMCID: PMC6473877.
235 Black DW, Grant JE, eds. *DSM-5 Guidebook: The Essential Companion to the Diagnostic and Statistical Manual of Mental Disorders, Fifth Edition*. Washington, DC: American Psychiatric, 2014.
236 Bishop TM, Walsh PG, Ashrafioun L, Lavigne JE, et al. "Sleep, suicide behaviors, and the protective role of sleep medicine." *Sleep Med*. 2020 Feb; 66: 264–70. doi: 10.1016/j.sleep.2019.07.016. Epub 2019 Jul 25.
237 Bishop TM, Crean HF, Hoff RA, Pigeon WR. "Suicidal ideation among recently returned veterans and its relationship to insomnia and depression." *Psychiatry Res*. 2019 Jun; 276: 250–261. doi: 10.1016/j.psychres.2019.05.019. Epub 2019 May 10.
238 Kecklund G, Axelsson J. "Health consequences of shift work and insufficient sleep." *BMJ*. 2016 Nov 1; 355: i5210. doi: 10.1136/bmj.i5210.
239 Kessler RC, Berglund PA, Coulouvrat C, Hajak G, et al. "Insomnia and the performance of US workers: Results from the America insomnia survey." *Sleep*. 2011 Sep 1; 34 (9): 1161–71. doi: 10.5665/SLEEP.1230.
240 Garbarino S, Magnavita N, Guglielmi O, Maestri M, et al. "Insomnia is associated with road accidents. Further evidence from a study on truck drivers." *PLoS One*. 2017 Oct 31; 12 (10): e0187256. doi: 10.1371/journal.pone.0187256. eCollection 2017.
241 McHill AW, Hull JT, Wang W, Czeisler CA, et al. "Chronic sleep curtailment, even without extended (>16-h) wakefulness, degrades human vigilance

performance." *Proc Natl Acad Sci U S A*. 2018 Jun 5; 115 (23): 6070–5. doi: 10.1073/pnas.1706694115. Epub 2018 May 21.

242 Söderström M, Jeding K, Ekstedt M, Perski A, et al. "Insufficient sleep predicts clinical burnout." *J Occup Health Psychol*. 2012 Apr; 17 (2): 175–83. doi: 10.1037/a0027518.

243 Elfering A, Kottwitz MU, Taman Ö, Müller U, et al. "Impaired sleep predicts onset of low back pain and burnout symptoms: Evidence from a three-wave study." *Psychol Health Med*. 2018 Dec; 23 (10): 1196–210. doi: 10.1080/13548506.2018.1479038. Epub 2018 May 24.

244 Spoken to Paul Begala during Clinton's 1992 campaign.

245 PTSD: National Center for PTSD. "2017 Clinical Practice Guideline for the Management of PTSD." U.S. Department of Veterans Affairs. 2020 Jan 30. Available at www.ptsd.va.gov/professional/treat/txessentials/cpg_ptsd_management.asp.

246 Roehrs T, Roth T. "Insomnia as a path to alcoholism: Tolerance development and dose escalation. *Sleep*. 2018 Aug 1; 41 (8): zsy091. doi: 10.1093/sleep/zsy091.

247 Chakravorty S, Chaudhary NS, Brower KJ. "Alcohol dependence and its relationship with insomnia and other sleep disorders." *Alcohol Clin Exp Res*. 2016 Nov; 40 (11): 2271–82. doi: 10.1111/acer.13217. Epub 2016 Oct 5.

248 Chakravorty S, Vandrey RG, He S, Stein MD. "Sleep management among patients with substance use disorders." *Med Clin North Am*. 2018 Jul; 102 (4): 733–43. doi: 10.1016/j.mcna.2018.02.012.

249 Ohayon MM. "Severe hot flashes are associated with chronic insomnia." *Arch Intern Med*. 2006 Jun 26; 166 (12): 1262–8. doi: 10.1001/archinte.166.12.1262.

250 Miner B, Gill TM, Yaggi HK, Redeker NS, et al. "Insomnia in community-living persons with advanced age." *J Am Geriatr Soc*. 2018 Aug; 66 (8): 1592–7. doi: 10.1111/jgs.15414. Epub 2018 May 21.

251 Vaz Fragoso CA, Gill TM. "Sleep complaints in community-living older persons: A multifactorial geriatric syndrome." *J Am Geriatr Soc*. 2007 Nov; 55 (11): 1853–66. doi: 10.1111/j.1532-5415.2007.01399.x. Epub 2007 Oct 3.

252 Patel D, Steinberg J, Patel P. "Insomnia in the elderly: A review." *J Clin Sleep Med*. 2018 Jun 15; 14 (6): 1017–24. doi: 10.5664/jcsm.7172.

253 Dopheide JA. "Insomnia overview: Epidemiology, pathophysiology, diagnosis and monitoring, and nonpharmacologic therapy." *Am J Manag Care*. 2020 Apr 12. 26: S76 S84. Available at www.ajmc.com/view/insomnia-overview-epidemiology-pathophysiology-diagnosis-and-monitoring-and-nonpharmacologic-therapy.

254 Liu MT. "Current and emerging therapies for insomnia." *Am J Manag Care*.

2020 Apr 12. 2020; 26: S85–S90. https://doi.org/10.37765/ajmc.2020. 43007 Introduction.

255 Gradisar M, Wolfson AR, Harvey AG, Hale L, et al. "The sleep and technology use of Americans: Findings from the National Sleep Foundation's 2011 Sleep in America poll." *J Clin Sleep Med*. 2013 Dec 15; 9 (12): 1291–9. doi: 10.5664/jcsm.3272.

256 LeBourgeois MK, Hale L, Chang A-M, Akacem LD, et al. "Digital media and sleep in childhood and adolescence." *Pediatrics*. 2017 Nov; 140 (Suppl 2): S92–6. doi: 10.1542/peds.2016-1758J.

257 Schutte-Rodin S, Broch L, Buysse D, Dorsey C, et al. "Clinical guideline for the evaluation and management of chronic insomnia in adults." *J Clin Sleep Med*. 2008 Oct 15; 4 (5): 487–504.

258 Sateia MJ, Buysse DJ, Krystal AD, Neubauer DN, et al. "Clinical practice guideline for the pharmacologic treatment of chronic insomnia in adults: An American Academy of Sleep Medicine clinical practice guideline." *J Clin Sleep Med*. 2017 Feb 15; 13 (2): 307–49. doi: 10.5664/jcsm.6470.

259 Harding EC, Franks NP, Wisden W. "The temperature dependence of sleep." *Front Neurosci*. 2019 Apr 24; 13: 336. doi: 10.3389/fnins.2019.00336.

260 Haghayegh S, Khoshnevis S, Smolensky MH, Diller KR, et al. "Before-bedtime passive body heating by warm shower or bath to improve sleep: A systematic review and meta-analysis." *Sleep Med Rev*. 2019 Aug; 46: 124–35. doi: 10.1016/j.smrv.2019.04.008. Epub 2019 Apr 19. PMID: 31102877.

261 Tordjman S, Chokron S, Delorme R, Charrier A, et al. "Melatonin: Pharmacology, functions and therapeutic benefits." *Curr Neuropharmacol*. 2017 Apr; 15 (3): 434–43. doi: 10.2174/1570159X14666161228122115. PMID: 28503116; PMCID: PMC5405617.

262 Saper CB, Fuller PM, Pedersen NP, Lu J, et al. "Sleep state switching." *Neuron*. 2010 Dec 22; 68 (6): 1023–42. doi: 10.1016/j.neuron.2010.11.032. PMID: 21172606; PMCID: PMC3026325.

263 Avallone R, Zanoli P, Corsi L, Cannazza G, et al. "Benzodiazepine compounds and GABA in flower heads of matricaria chamomilla." *Phytotherapy Res*. 1996; 10: 177–9.

264 Keefe JR, Mao JJ, Soeller I, Li QS, et al. "Short-term open-label chamomile (Matricaria chamomilla L.) therapy of moderate to severe generalized anxiety disorder." *Phytomedicine*. 2016 Dec 15; 23 (14): 1699–705. doi: 10.1016/j.phymed.2016.10.013. Epub 2016 Oct 24. PMID: 27912871; PMCID: PMC5589135.

265 Abdullahzadeh M, Matourypour P, Naji SA. "Investigation effect of oral chamomilla on sleep quality in elderly people in Isfahan: A randomized control trial." *J Educ Health Promot*. 2017 Jun 5; 6: 53. doi: 10.4103/jehp. jehp_109_15. PMID: 28616420; PMCID: PMC5470311.

266 Chang SM, Chen CH. "Effects of an intervention with drinking chamomile tea on sleep quality and depression in sleep disturbed postnatal women: A randomized controlled trial." *J Adv Nurs*. 2016 Feb; 72 (2): 306–15. doi: 10.1111/jan.12836. Epub 2015 Oct 20. PMID: 26483209.

267 Bent S, Padula A, Moore D, Patterson M, et al. "Valerian for sleep: A systematic review and meta-analysis." *Am J Med*. 2006; 119 (12): 1005–12. doi:10.1016/j.amjmed.2006.02.026. Available at www.ncbi.nlm.nih.gov/pmc/articles/PMC4394901.

268 Shinjyo N, Waddell G, Green J. "Valerian root in treating sleep problems and associated disorders-A systematic review and meta-analysis." *J Evid Based Integr Med*. 2020; 25: 2515690X20967323. doi:10.1177/2515690X20967323

269 Morin CM, Koetter U, Bastien C, Ware JC, et al. "Valerian-hops combination and diphenhydramine for treating insomnia: A randomized placebo-controlled clinical trial." *Sleep*. 2005 Nov; 28 (11): 1465–71. doi: 10.1093/sleep/28.11.1465. PMID: 16335333.

270 *Emser W, Bartylla K. "Improvement of sleep quality. Effect of kava extract WS 1490 on the sleep pattern in healthy subjects." Neurologie/Psychiatrie. 1991; 5 (11): 636–42.*

271 Ngan A, Conduit R. "A double-blind, placebo-controlled investigation of the effects of *Passiflora incarnata* (passionflower) herbal tea on subjective sleep quality." *Phytother Res*. 2011 Aug; 25 (8): 1153–9. doi: 10.1002/ptr.3400. Epub 2011 Feb 3. PMID: 21294203.

272 Guerrero FA, Medina GM. "Effect of a medicinal plant (*Passiflora incarnata* L) on sleep." *Sleep Sci*. 2017 Jul–Sep; 10 (3): 96–100. doi: 10.5935/1984-0063.20170018. PMID: 29410738; PMCID: PMC5699852.

273 Movafegh A, Alizadeh R, Hajimohamadi F, Esfehani F, et al. "Preoperative oral Passiflora incarnata reduces anxiety in ambulatory surgery patients: A double-blind, placebo-controlled study." *Anesth Analg*. 2008 Jun; 106 (6): 1728–32. doi: 10.1213/ane.0b013e318172c3f9. PMID: 18499602.

274 Koulivand PH, Khaleghi Ghadiri M, Gorji A. "Lavender and the nervous system." *Evid Based Complement Alternat Med*. 2013; 2013: 681304. doi: 10.1155/2013/681304. Epub 2013 Mar 14. PMID: 23573142; PMCID: PMC3612440.

275 Woelk H, Schläfke S. "A multi-center, double-blind, randomised study of the Lavender oil preparation Silexan in comparison to Lorazepam for generalized anxiety disorder." *Phytomedicine*. 2010 Feb; 17 (2): 94–9. doi: 10.1016/j.phymed.2009.10.006. Epub 2009 Dec 3. PMID: 19962288.

276 Conrad P, Adams C. "The effects of clinical aromatherapy for anxiety and depression in the high risk postpartum woman - a pilot study." *Complement Ther Clin Pract*. 2012 Aug; 18 (3): 164–8. doi: 10.1016/j.ctcp.2012.05.002. Epub 2012 Jun 27. PMID: 22789792.

277 Stilwell B. "NASA just researched the perfect nap." 2020 Apr 29. *We Are the Mighty.* Available at www.wearethemighty.com/mighty-culture/best-power-nap.

278 Tison GH, Avram R, Kuhar P, Abreau S, et al. "Worldwide effect of COVID-19 on physical activity: A descriptive study." *Ann Intern Med.* 2020 Nov 3; 173 (9): 767–70. doi: 10.7326/M20-2665. Epub 2020 Jun 29. PMID: 32598162; PMCID: PMC7384265.

279 DeFilippis E, Impink S, Singell M, Polzer JT, et al. "Collaborating during coronavirus: The impact of COVID-19 on the nature of work." Harvard Business School Organizational Behavior Unit Working Paper No. 21-006, Harvard Business School Strategy Unit Working Paper No. 21-006. 2020 Jul 16. Available at https://ssrn.com/abstract=3654470.

280 Tremblay A, Simoneau JA, Bouchard C. "Impact of exercise intensity on body fatness and skeletal muscle metabolism." *Metabolism.* 1994 Jul; 43 (7): 814–8. doi: 10.1016/0026-0495(94)90259-3. PMID: 8028502.

281 Viana RB, Naves JPA, Coswig VS, de Lira CAB, et al. "Is interval training the magic bullet for fat loss? A systematic review and meta-analysis comparing moderate-intensity continuous training with high-intensity interval training (HIIT)." *Br J Sports Med.* 2019 May; 53 (10): 655–64. doi: 10.1136/bjsports-2018-099928. Epub 2019 Feb 14. PMID: 30765340.

282 Boutcher SH. "High-intensity intermittent exercise and fat loss." *J Obes.* 2011; 2011: 868305. doi: 10.1155/2011/868305. Epub 2010 Nov 24. PMID: 21113312; PMCID: PMC2991639.

283 Kessler HS, Sisson SB, Short KR. "The potential for high-intensity interval training to reduce cardiometabolic disease risk." *Sports Med.* 2012 Jun 1; 42 (6): 489–509. doi: 10.2165/11630910-000000000-00000. PMID: 22587821.

284 Kravitz L. "Metabolic effects of HIIT." *IDEA Fitness Journal.* 2014. 11 (5): 16–8. Available at www.unm.edu/~lkravitz/Article%20folder/metabolicEffectsHIIT.html.

285 Craig BW, Brown R, Everhart J. "Effects of progressive resistance training on growth hormone and testosterone levels in young and elderly subjects." *Mech Ageing Dev.* 1989 Aug; 49 (2): 159–69. doi: 10.1016/0047-6374(89)90099-7. PMID: 2796409.

286 McPherron AC, Guo T, Bond ND, Gavrilova O. "Increasing muscle mass to improve metabolism." *Adipocyte.* 2013 Apr 1; 2 (2): 92–8. doi: 10.4161/adip.22500. PMID: 23805405; PMCID: PMC3661116.

287 Srikanthan P, Karlamangla AS. "Relative muscle mass is inversely associated with insulin resistance and prediabetes. Findings from the third National Health and Nutrition Examination Survey." *J Clin Endocrinol Metab.* 2011 Sep; 96 (9): 2898–903. doi: 10.1210/jc.2011-0435. Epub 2011 Jul 21. Erratum in: *J Clin Endocrinol Metab.* 2012 Jun;97(6):2203. PMID: 21778224.

288 Atlantis E, Martin SA, Haren MT, Taylor AW, et al; Members of the Florey Adelaide Male Ageing Study. "Inverse associations between muscle mass, strength, and the metabolic syndrome." *Metabolism.* 2009 Jul; 58 (7): 1013–22. doi: 10.1016/j.metabol.2009.02.027. PMID: 19394973.

289 Collins M, Renault V, Grobler LA, St Clair Gibson A, et al. "Athletes with exercise-associated fatigue have abnormally short muscle DNA telomeres." *Med Sci Sports Exerc.* 2003 Sep; 35 (9): 1524–8. doi: 10.1249/01. MSS.0000084522.14168.49. PMID: 12972872.

290 Urhausen A, Gabriel H, Kindermann W. "Blood hormones as markers of training stress and overtraining." *Sports Med.* 1995 Oct; 20 (4): 251–76. doi: 10.2165/00007256-199520040-00004. PMID: 8584849.

291 Tam CS, Johnson WD, Rood J, Heaton AL, et al. "Increased human growth hormone after oral consumption of an amino acid supplement: Results of a randomized, placebo-controlled, double-blind, crossover study in healthy subjects." *Am J Ther.* 2020 Jul/Aug; 27 (4): e333–7. doi: 10.1097/ MJT.0000000000000893. PMID: 30893070; PMCID: PMC6732240.

292 Casey A, Constantin-Teodosiu D, Howell S, Hultman E, et al. "Creatine ingestion favorably affects performance and muscle metabolism during maximal exercise in humans." *Am J Physiol.* 1996 Jul; 271 (1 Pt 1): E31–7. doi: 10.1152/ajpendo.1996.271.1.E31. PMID: 8760078.

293 Kreider RB, Ferreira M, Wilson M, Grindstaff P, et al. "Effects of creatine supplementation on body composition, strength, and sprint performance." *Med Sci Sports Exerc.* 1998 Jan; 30 (1): 73–82. doi: 10.1097/00005768-199801000-00011. PMID: 9475647.

294 Ross A, Thomas S. "The health benefits of yoga and exercise: A review of comparison studies." *J Altern Complement Med.* 2010 Jan; 16 (1): 3–12. doi: 10.1089/acm.2009.0044. PMID: 20105062.

295 Katuri KK, Dasari AB, Kurapati S, Vinnakota NR, et al. "Association of yoga practice and serum cortisol levels in chronic periodontitis patients with stress-related anxiety and depression." *J Int Soc Prev Community Dent.* 2016 Jan–Feb; 6 (1): 7–14. doi: 10.4103/2231-0762.175404. PMID: 27011926; PMCID: PMC4784068.

296 Michalsen A, Grossman P, Acil A, Langhorst J, et al. "Rapid stress reduction and anxiolysis among distressed women as a consequence of a three-month intensive yoga program." *Med Sci Monit.* 2005 Dec; 11 (12): CR55–561. Epub 2005 Nov 24. PMID: 16319785.

297 Vijayaraghava A, Doreswamy V, Narasipur OS, Kunnavil R, et al. "Effect of yoga practice on levels of inflammatory markers after moderate and strenuous exercise." *J Clin Diagn Res.* 2015 Jun; 9 (6): CC08–12. doi: 10.7860/ JCDR/2015/12851.6021. Epub 2015 Jun 1. PMID: 26266115; PMCID: PMC4525504.

298 Bharshankar JR, Bharshankar RN, Deshpande VN, Kaore SB, et al. "Effect

of yoga on cardiovascular system in subjects above 40 years." *Indian J Physiol Pharmacol.* 2003 Apr; 47 (2): 202–6. PMID: 15255625.

299 Yogendra J, Yogendra HJ, Ambardekar S, Lele RD, et al. "Beneficial effects of yoga lifestyle on reversibility of ischaemic heart disease: Caring heart project of International Board of Yoga." *J Assoc Physicians India.* 2004 Apr; 52: 283–9. PMID: 15636328.

300 Kolasinski SL, Garfinkel M, Tsai AG, Matz W, et al. "Iyengar yoga for treating symptoms of osteoarthritis of the knees: A pilot study." *J Altern Complement Med.* 2005 Aug; 11 (4): 689–93. doi: 10.1089/acm.2005.11.689. PMID: 16131293.

301 Farinatti PT, Rubini EC, Silva EB, Vanfraechem JH. "Flexibility of the elderly after one-year practice of yoga and calisthenics." *Int J Yoga Therap.* 2014; 24: 71–7. PMID: 25858653.

302 Tiedemann A, O'Rourke S, Sesto R, Sherrington C. "A 12-week Iyengar yoga program improved balance and mobility in older community-dwelling people: A pilot randomized controlled trial." *J Gerontol A Biol Sci Med Sci.* 2013 Sep; 68 (9): 1068–75. doi: 10.1093/gerona/glt087. Epub 2013 Jul 2. PMID: 23825035.

303 Lau C, Yu R, Woo J. "Effects of a 12-Week hatha yoga intervention on cardiorespiratory endurance, muscular strength and endurance, and flexibility in Hong Kong Chinese adults: A controlled clinical trial." *Evid Based Complement Alternat Med.* 2015; 2015: 958727. doi: 10.1155/2015/958727. Epub 2015 Jun 8. PMID: 26167196; PMCID: PMC4475706.

304 Bhutkar MV, Bhutkar PM, Taware GB, Surdi AD. "How effective is sun salutation in improving muscle strength, general body endurance and body composition?" *Asian J Sports Med.* 2011 Dec; 2 (4): 259–66. doi: 10.5812/asjsm.34742. PMID: 22375247; PMCID: PMC3289222.

305 Manjunath NK, Telles S. "Influence of yoga and ayurveda on self-rated sleep in a geriatric population." *Indian J Med Res.* 2005 May; 121 (5): 683–90. PMID: 15937373.

306 Harinath K, Malhotra AS, Pal K, Prasad R, et al. "Effects of Hatha yoga and Omkar meditation on cardiorespiratory performance, psychologic profile, and melatonin secretion." *J Altern Complement Med.* 2004 Apr; 10 (2): 261–8. doi: 10.1089/1075553043230622257. PMID: 15165407.

307 Birkel DA, Edgren L. "Hatha yoga: Improved vital capacity of college students." *Altern Ther Health Med.* 2000 Nov; 6 (6): 55–63. PMID: 11076447.

308 Sungkarat S, Boripuntakul S, Kumfu S, Lord SR, et al. "Tai chi improves cognition and plasma BDNF in older adults with mild cognitive impairment: A randomized controlled trial." *Neurorehabil Neural Repair.* 2018 Feb; 32 (2): 142–9. doi: 10.1177/1545968317753682. Epub 2018 Jan 20. PMID: 29353543.

309 Mortazavi H, Tabatabaeichehr M, Golestani A, Armat MR, et al. "The effect

of tai chi exercise on the risk and fear of falling in older adults: A randomized clinical trial." *Mater Sociomed*. 2018 Mar; 30 (1): 38–42. doi: 10.5455/msm.2018.30.38-42. PMID: 29670476; PMCID: PMC5857038.

310 Li F, Harmer P, Fitzgerald K, Eckstrom E, et al. "Tai chi and postural stability in patients with Parkinson's disease." *N Engl J Med*. 2012 Feb 9; 366 (6): 511–9. doi: 10.1056/NEJMoa1107911. PMID: 22316445; PMCID: PMC3285459.

311 Zheng S, Kim C, Lal S, Meier P, et al. "The effects of twelve weeks of tai chi practice on anxiety in stressed but healthy people compared to exercise and wait-list groups-A randomized controlled trial." *J Clin Psychol*. 2018 Jan; 74 (1): 83–92. doi: 10.1002/jclp.22482. Epub 2017 Jun 13. PMID: 28608523.

312 Chan AW, Yu DS, Choi KC, Lee DT, et al. "Tai chi qigong as a means to improve night-time sleep quality among older adults with cognitive impairment: A pilot randomized controlled trial." *Clin Interv Aging*. 2016 Sep 16; 11: 1277–86. doi: 10.2147/CIA.S111927. PMID: 27698557; PMCID: PMC5034925.

313 Wang C, Schmid CH, Hibberd PL, Kalish R, et al. "Tai Chi is effective in treating knee osteoarthritis: A randomized controlled trial." *Arthritis Rheum*. 2009 Nov 15; 61 (11): 1545–53. doi: 10.1002/art.24832. PMID: 19877092; PMCID: PMC3023169.

314 Wang C, Schmid CH, Iversen MD, Harvey WF, et al. "Comparative effectiveness of tai chi versus physical therapy for knee osteoarthritis: A randomized trial." *Ann Intern Med*. 2016 Jul 19; 165 (2): 77–86. doi: 10.7326/M15-2143. Epub 2016 May 17. PMID: 27183035; PMCID: PMC4960454.

315 Sanchez-Vazquez R, Guío-Carrión A, Zapatero-Gaviria A, Martínez P, et al. "Shorter telomere lengths in patients with severe COVID-19 disease." *Aging (Albany NY)*. 2021 Jan 11; 13 (1): 1–15. doi: 10.18632/aging.202463. Epub 2021 Jan 11. PMID: 33428591; PMCID: PMC7835063.

316 Marsa L. "Scientist of the Year Notable: Elizabeth Blackburn." *Discover Magazine*. 2007 Dec 6.

317 Slagboom PE, Droog S, Boomsma DI. "Genetic determination of telomere size in humans: A twin study of three age groups." *Am J Hum Genet*. 1994 Nov; 55 (5): 876–82. PMID: 7977349; PMCID: PMC1918314.

318 Huda N, Tanaka H, Herbert BS, Reed T, et al. "Shared environmental factors associated with telomere length maintenance in elderly male twins." *Aging Cell*. 2007 Oct; 6 (5): 709–13. doi: 10.1111/j.1474-9726.2007.00330.x. Epub 2007 Aug 24. PMID: 17725691.

319 Panossian LA, Porter VR, Valenzuela HF, Zhu X, et al. "Telomere shortening in T cells correlates with Alzheimer's disease status." *Neurobiol Aging*. 2003 Jan–Feb; 24 (1): 77–84. doi: 10.1016/s0197-4580(02)00043-x. PMID: 12493553.

320 Honig LS, Kang MS, Schupf N, Lee JH, et al. "Association of shorter leukocyte telomere repeat length with dementia and mortality." *Arch Neurol.* 2012 Oct; 69 (10): 1332–9. doi: 10.1001/archneurol.2012.1541. PMID: 22825311; PMCID: PMC3622729.

321 Minamino T, Miyauchi H, Yoshida T, Ishida Y, et al. "Endothelial cell senescence in human atherosclerosis: Role of telomere in endothelial dysfunction." *Circulation.* 2002 Apr 2; 105 (13): 1541–4. doi: 10.1161/01. cir.0000013836.85741.17. PMID: 11927518.

322 Fitzpatrick AL, Kronmal RA, Gardner JP, Psaty BM, et al. "Leukocyte telomere length and cardiovascular disease in the cardiovascular health study." *Am J Epidemiol.* 2007 Jan 1; 165 (1): 14–21. doi: 10.1093/aje/kwj346. Epub 2006 Oct 16. PMID: 17043079.

323 Brouilette S, Singh RK, Thompson JR, Goodall AH, et al. "White cell telomere length and risk of premature myocardial infarction." *Arterioscler Thromb Vasc Biol.* 2003 May 1; 23 (5): 842–6. doi: 10.1161/01. ATV.0000067426.96344.32. Epub 2003 Mar 20. PMID: 12649083.

324 von Zglinicki T, Serra V, Lorenz M, Saretzki G, et al. "Short telomeres in patients with vascular dementia: An indicator of low antioxidative capacity and a possible risk factor?" *Lab Invest.* 2000 Nov; 80 (11): 1739–47. doi: 10.1038/labinvest.3780184. PMID: 11092534.

325 Blasco MA. "Telomeres and cancer: A tale with many endings." *Curr Opin Genet Dev.* 2003 Feb; 13 (1): 70–6. doi: 10.1016/s0959-437x(02)00011-4. PMID: 12573438.

326 Cawthon RM, Smith KR, O'Brien E, Sivatchenko A, et al. "Association between telomere length in blood and mortality in people aged 60 years or older." *Lancet.* 2003 Feb 1; 361 (9355): 393–5. doi: 10.1016/S0140-6736(03)12384-7. PMID: 12573379.

327 Kitada T, Seki S, Kawakita N, Kuroki T, et al. "Telomere shortening in chronic liver diseases." *Biochem Biophys Res Commun.* 1995 Jun 6; 211 (1): 33–9. doi: 10.1006/bbrc.1995.1774. PMID: 7779103.

328 Harbo M, Bendix L, Bay-Jensen AC, Graakjaer J, et al. "The distribution pattern of critically short telomeres in human osteoarthritic knees." *Arthritis Res Ther.* 2012 Jan 18; 14 (1): R12. doi: 10.1186/ar3687. PMID: 22257826; PMCID: PMC3392801.

329 Zhai G, Aviv A, Hunter DJ, Hart DJ, et al. "Reduction of leucocyte telomere length in radiographic hand osteoarthritis: A population-based study." *Ann Rheum Dis.* 2006 Nov; 65 (11): 1444–8. doi: 10.1136/ard.2006.056903. Epub 2006 Oct 12. PMID: 17038452; PMCID: PMC1798337.

330 Saeed H, Abdallah BM, Ditzel N, Catala-Lehnen P, et al. "Telomerase-deficient mice exhibit bone loss owing to defects in osteoblasts and increased osteoclastogenesis by inflammatory microenvironment." *J Bone Miner Res.* 2011 Jul; 26 (7): 1494–505. doi: 10.1002/jbmr.349. PMID: 21308778.

NOTES

331 Valdes AM, Richards JB, Gardner JP, Swaminathan R, et al. "Telomere length in leukocytes correlates with bone mineral density and is shorter in women with osteoporosis." *Osteoporos Int.* 2007 Sep; 18 (9): 1203–10. doi: 10.1007/s00198-007-0357-5. Epub 2007 Mar 9. PMID: 17347788.

332 Kosmadaki MG, Gilchrest BA. "The role of telomeres in skin aging/photo-aging." *Micron.* 2004; 35 (3): 155–9. doi: 10.1016/j.micron.2003.11.002. PMID: 15036269.

333 Jackowska M, Hamer M, Carvalho LA, Erusalimsky JD, et al. "Short sleep duration is associated with shorter telomere length in healthy men: Findings from the Whitehall II Cohort Study." *PLoS One.* 2012; 7 (10): e47292. doi: 10.1371/journal.pone.0047292. Epub 2012 Oct 29. PMID: 23144701; PMCID: PMC3483149.

334 Prather AA, Puterman E, Lin J, O'Donovan A, et al. "Shorter leukocyte telomere length in midlife women with poor sleep quality." *J Aging Res.* 2011; 2011: 721390. doi: 10.4061/2011/721390. Epub 2011 Oct 20. PMID: 22046530; PMCID: PMC3199186.

335 Barceló A, Piérola J, López-Escribano H, de la Peña M, et al. "Telomere shortening in sleep apnea syndrome." *Respir Med.* 2010 Aug; 104 (8): 1225–9. doi: 10.1016/j.rmed.2010.03.025. Epub 2010 Apr 28. PMID: 20430605.

336 Pavanello S, Hoxha M, Dioni L, Bertazzi PA, et al. "Shortened telomeres in individuals with abuse in alcohol consumption." *Int J Cancer.* 2011 Aug 15; 129 (4): 983–92. doi: 10.1002/ijc.25999. Epub 2011 Apr 25. PMID: 21351086; PMCID: PMC3125427.

337 Bagnardi V, Rota M, Botteri E, Tramacere I, et al. "Light alcohol drinking and cancer: A meta-analysis." *Ann Oncol.* 2013 Feb; 24 (2): 301–8. doi: 10.1093/annonc/mds337. Epub 2012 Aug 21. PMID: 22910838.

338 Vachon CM, Cerhan JR, Vierkant RA, Sellers TA. "Investigation of an interaction of alcohol intake and family history on breast cancer risk in the Minnesota Breast Cancer Family Study." *Cancer.* 2001 Jul 15; 92 (2): 240–8. doi: 10.1002/1097-0142(20010715)92:2<240::aid-cncr1315>3.0.co;2-i. PMID: 11466675.

339 Chen WY, Rosner B, Hankinson SE, Colditz GA, et al. "Moderate alcohol consumption during adult life, drinking patterns, and breast cancer risk." *JAMA.* 2011 Nov 2; 306 (17): 1884–90. doi: 10.1001/jama.2011.1590. PMID: 22045766; PMCID: PMC3292347.

340 Kowalski S, Colantuoni E, Lau B, Keruly J, et al. "Alcohol consumption and CD4 T-cell count response among persons initiating antiretroviral therapy." *J Acquir Immune Defic Syndr.* 2012 Dec 1; 61 (4): 455–61. doi: 10.1097/QAI.0b013e3182712d39. PMID: 22955054; PMCID: PMC3541505.

341 Valdes AM, Andrew T, Gardner JP, Kimura M, et al. "Obesity, cigarette smoking, and telomere length in women." *Lancet.* 2005 Aug 20–26; 366 (9486): 662–4. doi: 10.1016/S0140-6736(05)66630-5. PMID: 16112303.

342 van der Vaart H, Postma DS, Timens W, ten Hacken NH. "Acute effects of cigarette smoke on inflammation and oxidative stress: A review." *Thorax*. 2004 Aug; 59 (8): 713–21. doi: 10.1136/thx.2003.012468. PMID: 15282395; PMCID: PMC1747102.

343 Wolkowitz OM, Mellon SH, Epel ES, Lin J, et al. "Leukocyte telomere length in major depression: Correlations with chronicity, inflammation and oxidative stress--preliminary findings." *PLoS One*. 2011 Mar 23; 6 (3): e17837. doi: 10.1371/journal.pone.0017837. PMID: 21448457; PMCID: PMC3063175.

344 Puterman E, Epel E. "An intricate dance: Life experience, multisystem resiliency, and rate of telomere decline throughout the lifespan." *Soc Personal Psychol Compass*. 2012 Nov 1; 6 (11): 807–25. doi: 10.1111/j.1751-9004.2012.00465.x. Epub 2012 Nov 5. PMID: 23162608; PMCID: PMC3496269.

345 Entringer S, Epel ES, Kumsta R, Lin J, et al. "Stress exposure in intrauterine life is associated with shorter telomere length in young adulthood." *Proc Natl Acad Sci U S A*. 2011 Aug 16; 108 (33): E513–8. doi: 10.1073/pnas.1107759108. Epub 2011 Aug 3. PMID: 21813766; PMCID: PMC3158153.

346 Harley C, Eppel E. Telomeres and Aging: how stress causes aging. TedMed Talk 2011.

347 Ornish D, Lin J, Daubenmier J, Weidner G, et al. "Increased telomerase activity and comprehensive lifestyle changes: A pilot study." *Lancet Oncol*. 2008 Nov; 9 (11): 1048–57. doi: 10.1016/S1470-2045(08)70234-1. Epub 2008 Sep 15. Erratum in: *Lancet Oncol*. 2008 Dec; 9 (12): 1124. PMID: 18799354.

348 Daubenmier J, Lin J, Blackburn E, Hecht FM, et al. "Changes in stress, eating, and metabolic factors are related to changes in telomerase activity in a randomized mindfulness intervention pilot study." *Psychoneuroendocrinology*. 2012 Jul; 37 (7): 917–28. doi: 10.1016/j.psyneuen.2011.10.008. Epub 2011 Dec 14. PMID: 22169588; PMCID: PMC3384690.

349 Lavretsky H, Epel ES, Siddarth P, Nazarian N, et al. "A pilot study of yogic meditation for family dementia caregivers with depressive symptoms: Effects on mental health, cognition, and telomerase activity." *Int J Geriatr Psychiatry*. 2013 Jan; 28 (1): 57–65. doi: 10.1002/gps.3790. Epub 2012 Mar 11. PMID: 22407663; PMCID: PMC3423469.

350 Jacobs TL, Epel ES, Lin J, Blackburn EH, et al. "Intensive meditation training, immune cell telomerase activity, and psychological mediators." *Psychoneuroendocrinology*. 2011 Jun; 36 (5): 664–81. doi: 10.1016/j.psyneuen.2010.09.010. Epub 2010 Oct 29. PMID: 21035949.

351 Rubin R. "As their numbers grow, COVID-19 'long haulers' stump experts." *JAMA*. 2020 Oct 13; 324 (14): 1381–3. doi: 10.1001/jama.2020.17709. PMID: 32965460.

352 Ricks D. *100 Questions & Answers about Coronaviruses.* Burlington, MA: Jones & Bartlett Learning, 2022.

353 Mokhtari T, Hassani F, Ghaffari N, Ebrahimi B, et al. "COVID-19 and multiorgan failure: A narrative review on potential mechanisms." *J Mol Histol.* 2020 Dec; 51 (6): 613–28. doi: 10.1007/s10735-020-09915-3. Epub 2020 Oct 4. PMID: 33011887; PMCID: PMC7533045.

354 Nugent J, Aklilu A, Yamamoto Y, Simonov M, et al. "Assessment of acute kidney injury and longitudinal kidney function after hospital discharge among patients with and without COVID-19." *JAMA Netw Open.* 2021 Mar 1; 4 (3): e211095. doi: 10.1001/jamanetworkopen.2021.1095. PMID: 33688965; PMCID: PMC7948062.

355 Sperati CJ. "Coronavirus: Kidney damage caused by COVID-19." Johns Hopkins University and Medicine. 2020 May 14. Available at www.hopkinsmedicine.org/health/conditions-and-diseases/coronavirus/coronavirus-kidney-damage-caused-by-covid19.

356 University Health Network. "Double-lung transplant after COVID-19 performed in Canada." University Health Network. 2021 Apr 12. Available at www.uhn.ca/corporate/News/Pages/Double_lung_transplant_after_COVID19_performed_in_Canada.aspx.

357 Nair P. "Profile of Shinya Yamanaka." *Proc Natl Acad Sci U S A.* 2012 Jun 12; 109 (24): 9223–5. doi: 10.1073/pnas.1121498109. Epub 2012 May 22. PMID: 22619323; PMCID: PMC3386100.

358 The Independent Panel for Pandemic Preparedness & Response. "Main Report & accompanying work." The Independent Panel for Pandemic Preparedness & Response. 2021 May. Available at https://theindependent-panel.org/mainreport.

359 Aschwanden C. "Five reasons why COVID herd immunity is probably impossible." *Nature.* 2021 Mar; 591 (7851): 520–2. doi: 10.1038/d41586-021-00728-2. PMID: 33737753.

360 McNeil Jr DG. "How much herd immunity is enough?" The New York Times. 2020 Dec 24. Available at www.nytimes.com/2020/12/24/health/herd-immunity-covid-coronavirus.html?smid=em-share.

361 Reguly E. "Why herd immunity to COVID-19 is proving elusive – even in highly vaccinated countries." The Globe and Mail. 2021 May 27. Available at www.theglobeandmail.com/world/article-herd-immunity-may-never-come-as-covid-19-variants-threaten-countries.

362 Oxford Reference. Available at www.oxfordreference.com/view/10.1093/oi/authority.20110803095750979#:~:text=adj.,endemic%20in%20Concise%20Medical%20Dictionary%20%C2%BB.

363 Phillips N. "The coronavirus is here to stay – here's what that means." *Nature.* 2021 Feb; 590 (7846): 382–4. doi: 10.1038/d41586-021-00396-2. PMID: 33594289.

364 Phillips N. "The coronavirus is here to stay – here's what that means." *Nature.* 2021 Feb; 590 (7846): 382–4. doi: 10.1038/d41586-021-00396-2. PMID: 33594289.

365 Centers for Disease Control and Prevention. "Weekly U.S. Influenza Surveillance Report." Centers for Disease Control and Prevention. Accessed 2021 May 31. Available at www.cdc.gov/flu/weekly/index.htm?web=1&wdLOR=cCC1F2C97-6E9B-394A-8A21-C7CBC004F69D.

366 Ritchie H, Ortiz-Ospina E, Beltekian D, Mathieu E, et al. "United Kingdom: Coronavirus Pandemic Country Profile." Our World in Data. Available at https://ourworldindata.org/coronavirus.

367 Centers for Disease Control and Prevention. "COVID Data Tracker Weekly Review." Centers for Disease Control and Prevention. Accessed 2021 May 31. Available at www.cdc.gov/coronavirus/2019-ncov/covid-data/covidview.

368 Valor Team. "Childhood trauma and addiction." Valor Recovery Centers. 2020 Feb 3. Available at www.valorrecoverycenters.com/recovery-reflections/childhood-trauma-and-addiction.

369 American Psychology Association. "One year later, a new wave of pandemic health concerns." American Psychology Association. 2021 Mar 11. Available at www.apa.org/news/press/releases/stress/2021/one-year-pandemic-stress.

370 Czeisler MÉ, Marynak K, Clarke KEN, Salah Z, et al. "Delay or avoidance of medical care because of COVID-19-related concerns - United States, June 2020." *MMWR Morb Mortal Wkly Rep.* 2020 Sep 11; 69 (36): 1250–7. doi: 10.15585/mmwr.mm6936a4. PMID: 32915166; PMCID: PMC7499838.

371 American Psychology Association. "One year later, a new wave of pandemic health concerns." 2021 Mar 11. American Psychology Association. Available at www.apa.org/news/press/releases/stress/2021/one-year-pandemic-stress.

372 Duhigg C. *The Power of Habit.* New York: Random House Books, 2014.

373 Graybiel AM. "Habits, rituals, and the evaluative brain." *Annu Rev Neurosci.* 2008; 31: 359–87. doi: 10.1146/annurev.neuro.29.051605.112851. PMID: 18558860.

374 Fogg BJ. "A Behavior Model for Persuasive Design." Stanford University. 2009 Apr 26. Available at www.implementation-hub.com/articles/A_Behavior_Model_for_Persuasive_Design.pdf.

375 Wood W, Neal DT. "A new look at habits and the habit-goal interface." *Psychol Rev.* 2007 Oct; 114 (4): 843–63. doi: 10.1037/0033-295X.114.4.843. PMID: 17907866.

376 Newland S. "The power of accountability." Association for Financial Counseling & Planning Education." 2018 3rd Quarter. Available at www.afcpe.org/news-and-publications/the-standard/2018-3/the-power-of-accountability.

377 Coelho P. *The Alchemist.* New York: HarperCollins, 2014.

NOTES

378 Grant A. "There's a name for the blah you're feeling: It's called languishing." The New York Times. 2021 Apr 19. Available at www.nytimes.com/2021/04/19/well/mind/covid-mental-health-languishing.html.
379 VanderWeele TJ. "On the promotion of human flourishing." *Proc Natl Acad Sci U S A*. 2017 Aug 1; 114 (31): 8148–56. doi: 10.1073/pnas.1702996114. Epub 2017 Jul 13. PMID: 28705870; PMCID: PMC5547610.
380 Winfrey O, Perry BD. *What Happened to You?* New York: Flatiron Books, 2021.
381 MetLife. "Redesigning the Employee Experience: Preparing the Workforce for a Transformed World," MetLife's 19th Annual U.S. Employee Benefit Trends Study 2021. Available at www.metlife.com/ebts2021.
382 World Health Organization. "Burn-out an 'occupational phenomenon': International Classification of Diseases." 2019 May 28. World Health Organization. Available at www.who.int/news/item/28-05-2019-burn-out-an-occupational-phenomenon-international-classification-of-diseases.
383 Innovation Health. "Why It's Critical to Develop a Vaccination Policy as Part of Your Overall Health And Safety Workplace Strategy." Innovation Health. 2021 May. Available at https://innovationhealthgroup.com/white-paper-1.
384 American Psychology Association. "One year later, a new wave of pandemic health concerns." American Psychology Association. 2021 Mar 11. Available at www.apa.org/news/press/releases/stress/2021/one-year-pandemic-stress.
385 Tollefson J. "COVID curbed carbon emissions in 2020 - but not by much." *Nature*. 2021 Jan; 589 (7842): 343. doi: 10.1038/d41586-021-00090-3. PMID: 33452515.
386 United Nations Environment Programme. "Cut global emissions by 7.6 percent every year for next decade to meet 1.5°C Paris target – UN report." United Nations Environment Programme. 2019 Nov 26. Available at www.unep.org/news-and-stories/press-release/cut-global-emissions-76-percent-every-year-next-decade-meet-15degc.
387 Kasotia P. "The health effects of global warming: Developing countries are the most vulnerable." United Nations. Accessed 2021 Jun 8. Available at www.un.org/en/chronicle/article/health-effects-global-warming-developing-countries-are-most-vulnerable.
388 Hill L, Popov J, Hartung E, Pai N. "Pediatric fecal microbiota transplantation for ulcerative colitis (PediFETCh): A preliminary report on feasibility." McMaster University. 2019 Mar 27. doi:10.13140/RG.2.2.35386.44481.